Aftermath in the ER

By Jimmy Hall

HAMMERTYME BOOKS

Dothan, Alabama

Aftermath in the ER

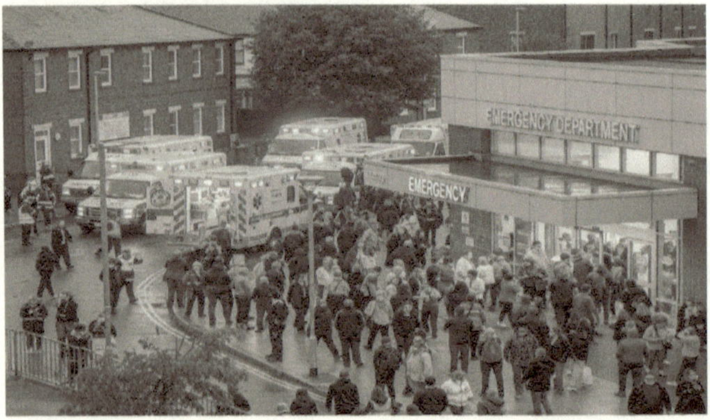

Photo: gemini.google.com

True Stories from the Frontlines of Emergency Medicine!

A memoir by Jimmy Hall.

In collaboration with emergency department nurses and physicians.

This is a non-fiction memoir. The stories in this book were transcribed from the memory of those who were personally interviewed. It reflects upon the recollection of experiences during the career of those involved. Some of the names, locations, and characteristics have been changed; some of the events have been compressed and portions of the dialogue have been recreated to protect the identity of some. Absolutely no patient or victim identifying information has been disclosed in this publication.

This book is presented for reading pleasure purposes only. While every attempt has been made to verify the information in this book, neither the author nor his affiliates assume any responsibility for errors, inaccuracies, or omissions.

Credits

Cover image from

https://www.freepik.com/author/wavebreakmedia-micro

HammerTyme Books Logo created by ChatGPT.

"https://www.ChatGPT.com"

Title Page & Section heading images created by:

http://gemini.google.com

Honorably Dedicated to:

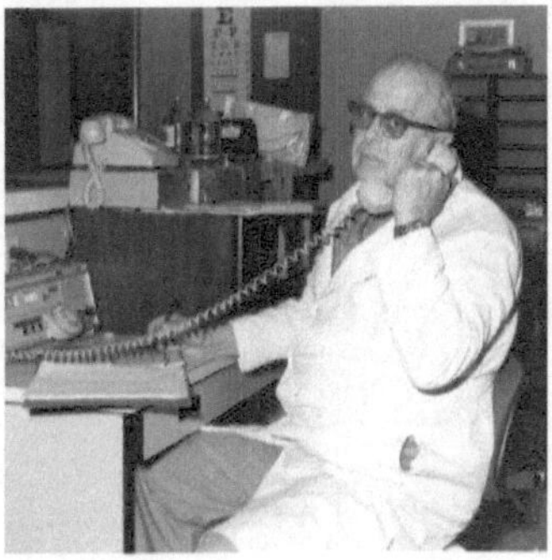

Dr. James M. Jones

June 8, 1925 – August 11, 1997

"A good doctor treats the disease; a great doctor treats the patient who has the disease." - William Osler

A truly exceptional ER physician and mentor—your dedication, skill, and compassion saved lives every day that you were present in the emergency department. In the face of chaos, you brought calm; in moments of crisis, you offered hope. Your tireless commitment and unwavering care made an immeasurable difference in the lives of your patients and the hearts of those who work alongside you in the trenches.

Thank you for being a healer, a leader, and an inspiration. Your presence has been greatly missed.

1 TABLE OF CONTENTS

INTRODUCTION

When I first wrote *Rekindled - True Stories of the Fire and EMS*, (Hall, 2025), I never anticipated the overwhelming response from readers. So many of you reached out, sharing how these stories resonated with your own experiences. That's when I knew I had to continue—there were still untold stories, still voices waiting to be heard. *Aftermath in the ER* follows the same gripping, heartfelt accounts from the front lines, but this time, I've shifted the focus from the streets to the heart of the emergency department.

Through the years, I have cherished the camaraderie and the privilege of sharing experiences with fellow fire service and EMS colleagues, ER nurses, and physicians. Reminiscing about the "good old days" not only strengthens our bonds but also preserves the rich history and culture of our profession.

As stories evolve over time, they take on a life of their own—seasoned by retellings, enriched by perspective. This natural progression keeps memories alive and engaging. To ensure these invaluable stories are not lost, we took on the task of documenting them—creating a lasting legacy for future generations. These accounts not only honor the past but also serve as a valuable resource for those stepping into the world of emergency medicine.

Aftermath in the ER, just like *Rekindled,* was created as a portal—a place where we can revisit these stories whenever we desire. More importantly, it serves as a vault, preserving them so they are never lost or forgotten. In doing so, we hope to contribute, in some small way, to the vital endeavor of historical preservation. By sharing these experiences, we aim to inspire, educate, and entertain those who dedicate their lives to emergency medicine.

This book is a compilation of true stories, as remembered by the ER nurses and physicians who stood on the front lines. Countless hours of interviews and conversations have gone into bringing these experiences to life. I sincerely thank you for purchasing your copy of *Aftermath in the ER*—I hope it brings back some of the most memorable moments of your career in the emergency department.

May God continue to bless you all and keep you safe!

The Gun & Knife Club

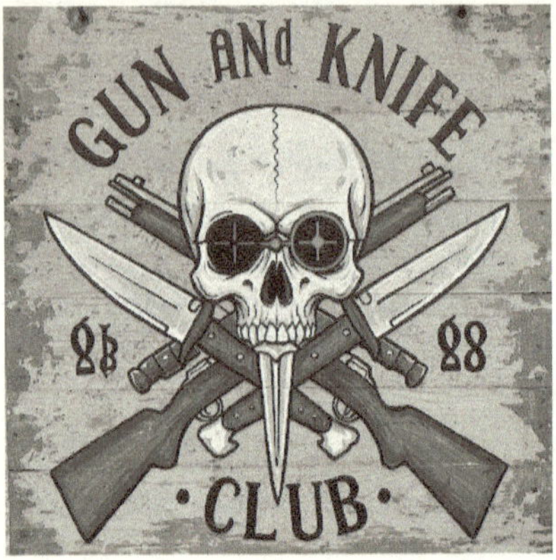

Photo: gemini.google.com

The emergency department has long been known by many names—ER, ED, trauma bay, the pit—but among seasoned emergency personnel, one of the most infamous monikers remains the "Gun and Knife Club." It's not a term you'll find on a nameplate or hospital directory, but it's whispered with a knowing smirk or a heavy sigh in break rooms and shift handoffs across the country. It's an unofficial title that speaks volumes about the raw, unfiltered reality of trauma care—the underbelly of emergency medicine where violence, unpredictability, and intensity collide.

The name itself may carry a tinge of dark humor, a coping mechanism that those in this profession understand all too well. It's a nod to the late-night arrivals of stabbing victims, the blaring of sirens announcing yet another gunshot wound, and the organized chaos of trauma resuscitations that unfold under flickering fluorescent lights. It represents the frontline of urban medicine, where clinicians don't just treat injuries—they run toward them.

For those who clock in each day (or more often, each night), the "Gun and Knife Club" isn't about morbidity—it's about reality. It's about knowing how to pack a wound while comforting a crying mother, how to keep a 17-year-old alive after a drive-by shooting while silently processing the tragedy of it all. It's about moving from one trauma bay to the next without missing a beat, adrenaline surging as you call out for blood products, chest tubes, or rapid sequence intubation—all while holding the line between life and death.

And yet, despite the brutality that often defines this corner of medicine, there is beauty here too. There's the synchronized ballet of a trauma team moving in perfect rhythm, the quiet strength of a nurse who's been through a hundred codes but still cares like it's their first, and the unspoken bond among colleagues forged in the fires of a shared crisis. It's a place where seasoned paramedics lay patients gently on gurneys, where nurses anticipate the next move before it's spoken, and where doctors whisper prayers as they push one more round of epinephrine.

Behind the sirens and statistics is a space filled with fierce compassion, technical brilliance, and emotional endurance. The "Gun and Knife Club," for all its darkness, is also a place where miracles happen—a place where the impossible sometimes becomes possible. It is here that the true spirit of emergency medicine reveals itself: not in the tragedy, but in the relentless hope, the hard-earned victories, and the unwavering commitment to fight for every heartbeat.

So while the name may be laced with gallows humor, it is also a badge of honor. It symbolizes a calling—a decision to stand in the gap when others turn away. And at the end of the longest shifts, after the stretchers have been cleared and the blood has been scrubbed away, what remains is a quiet pride in the knowledge that someone is still alive today... because of the work done in the club no one signs up for, but some are born to serve in.

"If You've Never Been There—Don't Speak on It" *by Amanda Caples, RN, Emergency Department / Dialysis*

As a former ICU nurse with years in acute dialysis, I thought I had seen it all. I've managed some of the most critically ill patients you can imagine. I've stood at the edge of life and death—advocating, acting fast, and pouring every ounce of skill and compassion into each decision.

But recently, I had the chance to work in the Emergency Department.

And let me tell you… it's a whole different world down there.

The pace is nonstop. The unpredictability is brutal. There's no time to think twice or lean on familiarity. ER nurses are triage experts, quick-thinking detectives, crisis negotiators, and lifesavers—sometimes all within a single minute. What looks like "just starting an IV" is often happening while juggling ten competing priorities in a loud, crowded room where the next door swing could mean *anything*.

And here's what I've learned—until you've been there, you don't fully understand. You might think you do—but assumptions aren't the same as experience.

Every department has its own pressure cooker. ICU, dialysis, ER—we each carry a version of controlled chaos. But no one is better than the other. We're just different gears in the same machine, all fighting to keep it moving.

Working across the hospital has taught me several things: *We should give each other more grace; Speak less judgement; Offer more understanding, because you never know the weight that someone is carrying.*

So the next time you feel tempted to criticize a unit you've never worked on, a shift you've never covered, or a role you've never played—pause.
Ask.
Learn.
Appreciate.

Because truthfully, we're all just showing up and giving the best we've got. And *that* deserves respect.

I'm so incredibly blessed to be doing what I was meant to do.

Amanda Caples, RN, Emergency Department / Dialysis

1 CHILDREN OF THE FOG

Early into my nursing career, I had a great opportunity to take on the role of the Emergency Department Nurse Director at Medical Center East. Early one morning I sat in the hospital's boardroom, with my focus split between the stack of compliance documents in front of me and the Joint Commission accreditation surveyor's probing questions. The JCAHO survey was a high-stakes evaluation, one that determined whether the hospital met national safety and quality standards.

The surveyor, Dr. John Stanley, a retired pediatrician, had just asked a question about the hospital's disaster preparedness when the boardroom phone buzzed urgently. One of the administrators, Brandon Jeffries, picked it up and then turned to me.

'Jimmy, it's for you.'

I rose to answer. The voice on the other end was my charge nurse, delivering a message I'll never forget—brief, but chilling:

"Code Black: EMS reporting 100+ pediatric patients inbound from a daycare center gas leak."

I immediately shot to my feet. "I have to go," I announced. "Mass casualty event—pediatric."

Dr. Stanley's eyebrows lifted in interest, and he immediately rose as well. "Do you mind if I observe?"

There was no time for formalities, I jerked my head toward the exit inviting him to follow me. We made our way swiftly to the ER, followed by the hospital administration team, where controlled chaos had already begun. Staff members moved with urgency, following the hospital's disaster protocol. The overhead speakers blared:

"Attention all staff: Code Black. MCI activation. Report to your designated department."

The first ambulance arrived within minutes. Directly behind it was a school bus with its flashing lights cutting through the morning fog underneath the ambulance bay. Children, ages three to five, spilled out, many coughing, their eyes red and watery. Paramedics rushed in to give quick status updates to the triage nurses, who categorized patients based on severity upon presentation.

Triage had been setup in the main ambulance entrance outside the ER. “Difficulty breathing goes to red zone!” shouted ER Charge Nurse Meghan Cole, as she began directing children with respiratory distress to ER bays. “Stable but symptomatic, yellow zone. Green tags to overflow.” Meghan continued.

The emergency department, already stretched on a normal day, had prepared for this scenario. Stretchers lined the hallways, additional ventilators were readied by the respiratory therapists, and the pediatric crash carts were pulled front and center.

A wave of nurses and physicians arrived after personnel recall messages were sent by the hospital. The other departments in the hospital also sent reinforcements to the personnel pool located in the hospital cafeteria. Respiratory therapists prepped nebulizers and oxygen masks. Social Workers grabbed stuffed animals to calm the frightened children.

I moved through the controlled mayhem, checking on my staff, overseeing the progress, and ensuring every child that presented to the emergency department received immediate care.

The next wave of patients arrived almost immediately with more children, some in mild distress, and others were somewhat lethargic. The ER was at capacity, but no child was left unattended. Every available hand was in motion—ER physicians, C-Suite staff, attending physicians, nurses, ER techs, ancillary staff, and even off-duty staff who had rushed back to help.

Lab techs processed blood gases and carboxyhemoglobin levels with astonishing speed. The pharmacy delivered medication and nebulized treatments. Social workers worked quickly to help reunite families.

Dr. Stanley, standing near the nurses' station, watched in awe. "I've done disaster preparedness surveys for years," he murmured to me as I juggled updates from EMS and the incident command center. "Never seen one play out in real time."

Three hours later, the worst was over. Not a single fatality. The gas exposure had been caught early, and every child was treated and stabilized. Families arrived in waves, clutching their little ones with relief.

As I finally exhaled, the weight of the chaos slowly lifting from my chest, I felt the sting of sweat beading on my forehead and trickling down my temples. My scrubs were damp, my back ached, and my hands—though steady—were beginning to feel the fatigue of everything they had done that day. The noise around me softened for just a moment, like the ER itself was catching its breath.

Through the fading hum of voices and the soft shuffle of post-incident cleanup, I saw Dr. Stanley approach. He wasn't in a hurry. His expression was calm, measured—like someone who had just witnessed something bigger than policy or protocol. There was a hint of humor in his eyes, the kind only a seasoned physician could wear after seeing the unthinkable unfold—and somehow resolve.

With his arms crossed and a subtle smirk tugging at the corners of his mouth, he nodded toward the controlled chaos behind me. “Well,” he said, with deliberate pause, “I was going to assess your ER disaster preparedness today…”

I blinked, already knowing where he was headed.

“…but I don’t think that’ll be necessary,” he finished. “I have my answer.”

Despite the exhaustion dragging at my limbs, I chuckled—dry, breathless, but real. “And?”

He stepped closer, extended his hand with genuine respect, and said the words I didn’t realize I needed to hear.

“You passed.”

A wave of emotion rose in my chest—relief, pride, and that strange mix of adrenaline and gratitude that only comes when you know lives were saved because you didn’t break. Around us, the team—still catching their own breath—let out a round of tired but triumphant cheers. Some clapped, others fist-bumped or simply nodded in solidarity. We didn’t need a formal announcement. We knew.

We had been tested—not with drills or scenarios, but with real patients, real decisions, and real consequences. And somehow, against the odds, we had risen to the moment. Together.

Medical Center East was ready. Not because we were perfect, but because when everything hit the fan—we stood our ground, side by side.

And today, because of that... many children got to go home.

Alive.

Safe.

Because we were ready when it counted.

2 STOP, DROP, AND BOUNCE

It was a warm day in the midmorning when the emergency department doors swung open, and a frantic man rushed in, exclaiming in broken English that his wife was having a baby. The nurse on duty, Angela Smith, grabbed a wheelchair and hurried to the ambulance entrance, where a battered old van had just pulled up.

As Angela reached the van, she saw a young Latina woman, her face glimmering with sweat, breathing heavily, with an extremely noticeable bulge in her pants that made Angela's heart race. With quick but gentle movements, she helped the woman into the wheelchair and pushed her toward an open ER bay.

As soon as the patient was settled on the bed, Angela and another nurse, Liz, carefully removed the woman's pants. To their astonishment, nestled between her legs was a full-term baby boy, still attached to the umbilical cord. His tiny chest rose and fell steadily, his skin a healthy pink. He was quiet but alert.

Angela swiftly assessed the newborn, performing an APGAR test. The baby was strong and healthy. The doctor on call, Dr. Edward Kristi, entered the room with practiced efficiency, donning gloves and preparing to cut the umbilical cord and deliver the placenta.

Meanwhile, the mother, still catching her breath, suddenly blurted out, "Work! Work! Work!" Her voice was urgent, her dark eyes filled with worry.

Dr. Kristi shook his head. "No, you need to stay here. You just gave birth to a baby. We have to deliver the placenta and make sure you're okay."

Despite her protests, the medical team proceeded with the necessary care. The placenta was delivered without any complications, and both the mother and the baby were cleaned and wrapped in warm blankets. The woman held her son briefly, staring down at his face, her expression unreadable. Then, she looked at the clock on the wall.

"Work," she whispered again, almost pleading.

Angela sighed and placed a gentle hand on the woman's shoulder. "You need to rest. Your body has been through a lot today. You need to stay here until you're fully recovered."

The woman nodded, but something in her demeanor seemed restless. Not long afterward, Angela stepped out to retrieve her chart. When she returned, the mother was not in the room. The crib still held the swaddled newborn, but the mother and her family member had vanished.

A search ensued. Security scoured the hospital, checking hallways and exits, but she was nowhere to be found. The local police were called, but their search of the surrounding area yielded nothing.

Then a phone call was made by the social worker to the patient's employer which was listed in her medical records. The employer at the tomato farm confirmed what the hospital staff had feared all along—she had left the hospital and returned to work.

DHR was contacted, and an assessment was made. The mother insisted she wanted her child and assured them she would return to retrieve him when her shift ended.

The hospital staff exchanged troubled glances. A woman who had just given birth, who had not yet fully recovered, was back in the grueling heat of the fields. The strength and resilience of this woman was undeniable, but the weight of her circumstances was just as stark.

The newborn remained in the hospital nursery until he was ready for discharge by the pediatrician. The mother came for the child......but not until after her shift had ended.

3 When Angels Cry

This story is based on a true event, with the names and specific details altered to protect those involved. While some elements have been changed, the message remains the same.

The sun had barely begun to rise one morning when Henry Harrison stepped onto his front porch, his steaming cup of coffee in hand. He took a deep breath of the crisp morning air, expecting to hear the familiar sound of tiny feet scampering about. Every morning on her way to work, Henry's daughter would drop off his grandson for the day with his grandparents while she worked. Without fail, each morning, this four-year-old grandson, Cole, would rush to him, eyes bright with excitement, ready for their daily ritual of feeding the ducks down by the pond. But today, there was only silence.

Henry's heart clenched because it was very unusual for Cole to stray away from routine. He set his coffee down, calling out for Cole. No answer. Panic creeping into his chest, he searched the house, checking every room, then hurried outside, scanning the yard. Still nothing. Then, his eyes drifted toward the pond.

With growing dread, Henry hurried down to the pier, his boots thudding against the wooden planks. His breath caught in his throat when he saw it—a small, overturned container of duck feed spilling its contents onto the worn boards. His gaze shifted to the water, and what he saw made his knees buckle.

There, at the bottom of the pond, was Cole.

Henry's frantic shouts shattered the morning calm as he scrambled into the water, his aged limbs moving with desperation. He pulled the boy's limp body to the surface and onto the pier, his own breath coming in ragged gasps. He shook him, called his name, pressed against his tiny chest, but there was no response. His skin was cold, his lips tinged a deep blue.

With trembling fingers, Henry fumbled for his phone, his voice breaking as he called 911. Within minutes, the wail of sirens filled the air, and the EMS team rushed in. "Code Pink," one of them called out. Pediatric Advanced Life Support protocol was initiated, hands working feverishly to restart the little heart. Cole was swiftly transported to the emergency department, where the hospital team took over the fight for his life.

Doctors and nurses surrounded him, each second precious, and each movement urgent. His body remained still, unresponsive. The monitors were silent, and after over an hour of relentless efforts, the team had to face the unbearable truth.

There was nothing more they could do.

The room fell into a heavy silence as the team stepped back, sorrow weighing on their shoulders.

Cole's body was gently cleaned and prepared, wrapped in a soft white blanket by his nurses. He was moved upstairs to a quiet room on the pediatric floor, where his grieving family had gathered. His mother, shattered and hollow-eyed, took her little boy into her arms, rocking him as she had done countless times before, whispering to him softly through her sobs.

In the midst of their sorrow, a glimmer of hope emerged when the hospital's nurse supervisor gently approached them about organ donation. Maybe, just maybe, Cole could help another child live. But that fragile hope was soon crushed—the prolonged time in the water had made him ineligible for any type of donation.

The loss felt even greater.

As the family sat in their silent grief, the ER Nurse Director, who also worked per diem for the state eye bank, came forward. He carried with him a book, *The Nicholas Effect,* by Reg Green —a true story about a child in Europe who had donated his organs after a tragic event that took his life. It was a small offering, a gesture of comfort in their darkest hour. Cole's parents clung to it, grateful for something—anything—to hold onto.

Months later, on a somber afternoon, Cole's mother and grandmother returned to the ER. In their hands, they carried a framed portrait of the little boy. They placed it gently on the counter of the nurse's station, looking up at the nurses and doctors with tearful gratitude.

"I wanted you all to see what he really looked like," Cole's mother said, her voice trembling. "When he was alive. When he was full of spirit."

Not a single eye remained dry that day. Not in that moment—not on the tragic day when the ER team had fought so hard for a little boy whose only desire was to simply feed the ducks.

Losing a child in the ER is one of the most heartbreaking experiences a medical team can face. Despite every effort, every skill, and every ounce of determination, sometimes the outcome is out of their hands. The weight of that loss lingers—felt in the silence after the chaos, in the eyes of grieving parents, and in the hearts of the team who fought so very hard to save a life that was far too young to go. It's a tragedy that never gets easier, a sorrow that stays with those who dedicate their lives to healing forever.

4 God Doesn't Like Ugly

It was an Easter Sunday in the emergency department that wasn't any different from any other holiday—chaotic yet oddly slow in stretches. Dr. Drayton Barker, one of the hospital's top neurosurgeons, sat at the nurses' station, charting notes on a consult he had just finished. He had little patience for small talk, especially when it turned to religious beliefs.

At the edge of his consciousness, he heard a gaggle of nurses chatting between the annoying sound of patient call lights and IV beeps. Their conversation had shifted from chocolate bunnies and egg hunts to something more solemn.

"I just can't imagine what Jesus endured on the cross," Nichole murmured.

"It's incredible, really. The suffering, the humility, the sacrifice—it hurts my heart just thinking about it," Janie added.

Dr. Barker scoffed, shaking his head. He had spent his career inside the human brain, unraveling its mysteries, repairing its injuries.

Science, skill, and logic dictated his world—not faith, not fairy tales. He had no patience for sentimental musings about a man who had died two thousand years ago.

Shoving his chair back, he stood and turned to the nurses. *"I don't know what it is that you find so fascinating about all that God stuff,"* he said, his voice dripping with condescension. Without another word, he strode out of the nurse's station, his white coat billowing behind him.

Then, just as he rounded the corner of the desk—

His feet shot out from under him as if pulled by an unseen force. He didn't even have time to catch himself. His head hit the cold hard floor first with a sickening *crack*. A jolt of white-hot pain surged through his skull.

A stunned silence fell over the nurses' station.

Dr. Barker scrambled to his feet, his face pale, his eyes wide with something between shock and fear. Without a word, he adjusted his coat and rushed out of the emergency department, disappearing down the hall.

The nurses exchanged bewildered glances before hurrying over to inspect the floor. They expected to find spilled water, a stray IV bag, something—anything—that could explain what had just happened.

But the floor was bone dry. There was no slick surface, no obstruction. Nothing.

Pam swallowed hard and whispered, *"Well... that's interesting."*

Janie, still staring at the pristine floor, murmured, *"He might not believe in God... but it looks like someone believes in him."*

And with that, they returned to their work, a silent reverence settling over them—because some things, even in a hospital filled with science and reason, defied explanation.

5 COLLATERAL DAMAGE

The emergency department was bustling with the usual chaos of an understaffed, overworked Sunday shift. Among the controlled madness, a new patient checked in—a middle-aged IV drug abusing woman with a swollen, angry abscess on her forearm. The thing was ripe, red, and pulsating like it had a heartbeat of its own.

Dr. Franklin Meriwether, a notoriously unreserved physician, spotted the case on the board and saw an opportunity—not just for medicine, but for a little showmanship. Dr. Meriwether loved to teach, especially when it included the fresh-faced nursing students who hung on his every word.

"Who wants in on an I&D?" he called out, grinning.

The students perked up immediately. "Absolutely!" one of them beamed.

Even some of the staff nurses, particularly the ones who took an odd satisfaction in squeezing pus, angled for a spot in the makeshift surgical theater behind the curtain. But who was the lucky nurse assigned to the patient? None other than me, I despised abscesses more than anything.

"Anyone want to trade?" I asked, looking around. "I'll take literally anything else."

Before I could finish my plea, Sarah, one of the more enthusiastic nurses, practically jumped at the offer. "I'll trade! I got a Foley Cath on an elderly man."

I narrowed my eyes and said. "You serious?"

Sarah crossed her arms. "Dead serious."

I sighed, but out of relief instead of despair. "Deal."

While Sarah gleefully joined the abscess extraction team, I walked over to see my new patient, relieved to be spared the impending flood of pus. But just as I finished setting up for the catheter, a commotion erupted from behind the curtain where the I&D was happening.

It started with a single shriek. Then another. And then—pure pandemonium.

Like a herd of panicked cattle, the entire group burst from behind the curtain, tripping over each other, eyes wide with horror. Some were gagging, others were dry-heaving, and a few were bolting for the nearest sink. The foulest, most putrid stench imaginable rolled across the ER like the breath from a demonic dragon.

A tech staggered out, holding his head. "It—oh God—it hit the ceiling!"

Dr. Meriwether stumbled out next, his pristine white coat now a canvas of brownish-yellow icing. His once-confident smirk had vanished, replaced by an expression of pure regret.

The students? Traumatized. At least one of them was leaning against a wall, clutching their stomach.

The nurses who had *begged* to be in there? They were now paying the price, retching in unison.

I myself, however, simply grinned. I adjusted my gloves, patted my elderly patient on the shoulder, and said, "Now, this is why you always trade smart."

And with that, I got back to work—completely unscathed. Sometimes it works out in your favor when you work smart.

After everyone had settled back down and the emergency department had returned to a near-normal level, I overheard Sarah asking Jill, another ER nurse—"How do you write *the abscess was very pus-sy?*" I shook my head and moved on.

6 Raw Head & Bloody Bones

It was just after 8 a.m. when the radio buzzed over the emergency department speaker. Marilyn McKissack, the ER Director, sipped her coffee and listened intently from the nurse's station as the voice on the line relayed an incoming trauma alert.

"38 Mary 10 is enroute with a male patient, approximately 60 years old. Multiple extremity injuries—upper and lower. Patient reportedly fell off his tractor and was mauled by a bush hog. Significant open wounds, fractures, and partial amputations to arms and legs. Vitals stable for now. ETA 5 minutes."

Heads turned. Bush hog injuries weren't unheard of in South Alabama, but they were always messy, always ugly, and always *very* serious.

Marilyn snapped into action, directing staff to prep Trauma Room 2, notify surgery, and clear the hallway. The team moved fast—IV carts rolled in, blood bank was notified, monitors were ready, and the trauma team stood waiting as the sirens approached.

The ambulance backed into the bay, the doors opened to reveal the mangled patient, his arms and legs lacerated and fractured from the tremendous power of the bush hog. His coveralls were soaked in blood, bits of denim and flesh torn away. The medics gave report as the team quickly transferred him to the trauma bed, swarming like bees—cutting clothes, starting lines, stabilizing fractures, and controlling bleeding.

He was whisked away to surgery within minutes, a coordinated ballet of speed and expertise.

As the tension broke and the adrenaline slowly faded, Marilyn stood at the edge of the nurse's station, shaking her head solemnly.

"Lord have mercy," she said. "Can you even imagine being attacked by such a vicious animal?"

Silence.

Every single person in the room froze and slowly turned to face her.

"Wait," Steve Hartman said carefully. "What do you mean *animal*?"

Marilyn looked around, eyes wide. "The bush hog," she said, completely serious. "That wild thing that attacked him... I mean, how big are they? Do they travel in packs?"

There it was. A full three-second pause. Time truly stopped.

Then—*boom*—the room exploded in laughter.

One of the medics grabbed a chair to keep from falling over. One of the techs clapped his hands and bent over wheezing. Even Dr. Jones, the ER Medical Director, had to step out of the trauma bay to regain composure.

"You mean to tell me," Dr. Jones said between gasps, "you thought the man got mauled by a *wild animal called a Bush Hog*?!"

Marilyn blinked. "Wait... Bush Hog isn't an animal?"

That was it. The final straw. People collapsed into chairs, nurses wiped tears from their eyes, and even the trauma surgeon was told mid-surgery: *Marilyn McKissack thinks a Bush Hog is a rabid farm beast.*

Within hours, the name stuck like duct tape.

Dr. Jones—never one to let a good nickname die—started referring to her exclusively as *Bush Hog* over the intercom.

"Bush Hog to triage... Bush Hog, your lunch is at the desk..."

A few days later, Marilyn entered the ER break room to find a giant laminated poster taped to the refrigerator. It was a feral-looking razorback hog with glowing red eyes and the caption:

"South Alabama's Most Feared Predator — *The Bush Hog*"

Rumor had it, the cardiologist, Sawyer Jameson, had the poster printed at the local sign shop. And Marilyn? She took it like a champ—half-blushing, half-laughing every time someone brought it up, which was often.

To this day, whether you work days, nights, or PRN, you don't mention "Marilyn McKissack" without someone replying, “Oh, you mean *Bush Hog*?”

Because in emergency medicine, the moments that save lives might make the headlines…

…but the moments that *make legends* always start with a good laugh.

7 THE MYSTERIOUS CARROT

It was a relatively calm day in the ER—well, as calm as any ER ever gets—when the ER registration clerk called over the intercom: *"We've got a walk-in... complaint of rectal pain... says he has a foreign object lodged in his rectum."*

Heads turned. Every nurse, tech, and doc in earshot knew what that meant. Foreign body extractions were always interesting.

When the patient was brought back to a room, the attending physician, Dr. William Boyd, took a deep breath before pulling back the curtain. Lying on the bed was a middle-aged man, shifting uncomfortably and looking like he wished he were anywhere else.

"Sir, can you tell me what brings you in today?"

The man hesitated, cleared his throat, and then finally muttered, *"There's... a whole carrot... in my butt."*

Dr. Boyd blinked. "A whole carrot?"

The man nodded solemnly.

Now, ER docs have heard it all, but protocol still requires asking how these objects end up where they do. So, with his best poker face, Dr. Boyd asked, *"Can you explain to me how this happened?"*

The man sat up a little, wincing as he did. *"I was unloading groceries from my car. I tripped. I fell. Right onto a bag. One of the carrots must've, uh, shot up there."*

There was a moment of silence. Then Dr. Boyd, unable to stop himself, raised an eyebrow. *"Through your pants?"*

The man turned bright red. *"...Yes."*

The attending nurse nearly choked on her own breath.

An X-ray confirmed the man was telling the *partial* truth—there was indeed a carrot lodged where carrots were never meant to go. But how it got there? Well, that was between him and his skewed imagination.

Surgery was called, and the OR team prepared for yet another round of foreign-object retrieval. The surgeon, Dr. Charles O'Conner, after hearing the story, sighed and muttered, *"Why is it always vegetables?"*

As the patient was wheeled off to the OR, Dr. Boyd turned to the nurse and said, *"Salad bar for dinner?"*

Another day, another ER legend in the making.

8 Shocking Attitude Adjustment

It was already shaping up to be, yet again, one of those nights in the ER—you know, the kind where the full moon must be out, even if the calendar says otherwise. The Big Phone rang and the charge nurse made the announcement:

"We've got EMS bringing in a combative prisoner with PD escort. Head laceration. Unruly. Buckle up, guys."

A few sighs and eye-rolls followed because everyone knew what that meant. The ER staff had long accepted that patching up rowdy drunks and belligerent troublemakers was just part of the job description.

Minutes later, EMS, along with two uniformed officers rolled in, escorting a man who looked like he'd had a rough night. His face was smeared with dried blood from a gash on his forehead, his shirt was torn, and he was fuming mad.

"I don't need no damn doctor!" the man barked, yanking against the handcuffs that were secured in front of him. *"You people just wanna mess with me!"*

Dr. Pete Vickers, the ER physician, had seen it all. He approached the man with his usual calm, professional demeanor.

"Sir, I need to check that wound before it gets worse. Can you cooperate so I can help you?"

The prisoner scoffed. *"Man, get outta my face with that! You ain't touching me!"*

The two officers exchanged glances. One of them, a veteran cop, sighed like this was far from his first rodeo with this particular character.

Dr. Vickers tried again, but the patient kept thrashing, cursing, and flailing just enough to make any attempt at medical care impossible. Finally, after almost getting a wayward loogie projectile to the shoulder, Dr. Vickers threw up his hands.

"Alright, you don't want help? Fine. But you're not going to sit here and make it impossible for us to do our jobs."

That's when it happened.

The man suddenly hopped off the foot of the stretcher and started walking—no, storming—toward the exit still in handcuffs. The two cops stiffened, and one immediately commanded, *"Hey man! Stop right there!"*

But the man kept going, not a care in the world.

Pop!

Followed by the unmistakable *ZZZZZZZZZT* of a Taser deployment.

The man froze mid-step like someone had just hit the pause button on his life, then *WHOMP!*—he hit the tile floor like a freshly chopped tree.

Everyone in the ER turned to look. Silence. Then... twitching.

The cops, ever efficient, walked over, picked him up off the floor like a sack of potatoes, and plopped him right back onto the stretcher.

The man blinked, clearly trying to process what had just happened. He looked at Dr. Vickers, his attitude now completely different.

"Sir," he said, his voice shaking slightly, *"I am so very sorry for acting like I did. Please, do whatever you need to do to help me. I will not be any further problem."*

Dr. Vickers smiled, nodded, and grabbed his suture tray.

It is amazing how a little jolt of electricity can quickly change a bad attitude.

9 Catch and Release

A crazy start to a "Q-word" morning in the ER—increased ambulance calls, flu cases, GI complaints. But nothing could have prepared the staff for what was about to come through the doors.

The triage desk was fairly calm when a man in his mid-30s staggered in, hunched over, gripping the front of his jeans like he was holding on for dear life. His face was beet red, and he was sweating bullets.

I was the triage nurse. I greeted the patient and I barely had time to ask *"What brings you in today?"* before the man groaned through gritted teeth:

"I... my... my JUNK is stuck in my ZIPPER!"

There was a pause. I blinked, I looked, and then, without another word, I grabbed the chart, stood up, and motioned for the man to follow me. I walked through the triage doors into the emergency department, guiding the patient with a sense of urgency in my stride. We made our way to Bay 3, my focus sharp. Later, my female coworkers couldn't wait to share with me just how comical they found my actions to be.

Jeanne Emrick, RN, laughed as she remembered, *"He emerged from triage like a man on a mission!"*

"Jimmy's voice cut through the usual ER chatter: Room 3! NOW! Jeanne—get the doctor, STAT!" Jeanne said while continuing to giggle.

Jeanne, a veteran ER nurse who had seen just about everything, looked up from her paperwork. *"Is he coding?"* she called after him.

I think I shot her a look and said. *"Just get the doc!"*

Within seconds, Dr. Tim Adamcryk and veteran ER nurse, Robert Smith, rushed into Room 3, finding the patient already lying on the stretcher, his pants still half-zipped, agony written all over his face. I was already in action, pulling up a syringe filled with lidocaine.

Jeanne peered through the curtain and later recalled that it was *the fastest she had ever seen those three work in her entire career*. It was as if the man's life was on the line—except, in a way, his dignity certainly was.

As Dr. Adamcryk assessed the situation, he let out a low whistle. *"That's... quite a predicament."*

I didn't hesitate. *"I'm injecting lidocaine now."*

The patient groaned. *"Please, just get it out! I was sitting on the toilet when my brother showed up to take me fishing. I jumped up, no underwear, zipped too fast, and—"* He winced, unable to finish the sentence.

Dr. Adamcryk, Robert, and I all three collectively felt *phantom pain* just hearing it.

With the area numbed as much as possible, Dr. Adamcryk grabbed a pair of medic shears, while Robert and I carefully maneuvered the zipper with hemostats, then pliers. *Snip. Tug. Wiggle.*

Then finally—**freedom!**

The patient let out a deep, shaky breath of relief.

"You guys," he mumbled, *"are lifesavers."*

Robert grinned. *"Next time, buddy... wear some underwear."*

To this day, Jeanne still brings up that incident, laughing about how it almost looked like a cardiac arrest case the way those guys sprang into action.

10 URINE SAMPLE TASTE TEST

Mixie Becker was a force to be reckoned with in the ER—very skillful with her hands, quicker with her wit, and known throughout the hospital for her legendary pranks. If you were new to the emergency room, it was only a matter of time before you became a victim of one of her well-orchestrated shenanigans.

Her favorite? The "urine taste test."

Whenever a group of nursing students were assigned to the ER, Mixie would pull one of her colleagues aside—which in many cases was me, her routine partner-in-crime—and set the prank in motion.

"Hey, Jimmy, I need a urine sample on Mr. Peterson in room five," she'd say with a perfectly straight face.

Because I was already in on the joke, I would take a specimen cup, fill it with apple juice, and return it to her in front of the unsuspecting students. Mixie would then remove the lid, dip her finger into the golden liquid, put it in her mouth, and make a thoughtful expression.

"Uhhhh, that's a little sweet," she'd announce, smacking her lips for dramatic effect. "Better send this one to the lab for further analysis."

Without fail, the students' faces would twist into expressions of pure horror, some turning green, others backing away in shock. Mixie and I would hold our composure just long enough before bursting into laughter, letting the poor students in on the joke.

One day, after pulling off another successful round of pranks, I leaned in, still chuckling. "Hey Mixie," I said, with my eyes twinkling with mischief, "what if I actually put real urine in the cup and handed it to you?"

Mixie didn't miss a beat. She shot me a deadly serious look, one eyebrow arched, and said, "Jimmy, I would kill you."

I burst into laughter again, but deep down, I knew better than to test Mixie Becker. She might've been the queen of pranks—but cross her, and you might just find yourself on the receiving end of one of her pranks that you'd never forget.

11 WINTER DAY MIRACLE

It was an unusually cold winter day in the South when Mr. Charles Jones collapsed. He had been outside working when a sharp pain radiated across his chest. Recognizing the symptoms, he sent one of his workers, Ezekiel Harris, to fetch his nitroglycerin pills. But by the time he had returned, Mr. Jones was unconscious, his breath stilled, his heartbeat silent.

Panic surged among all the workers, but Ezekiel, though untrained in CPR, refused to stand idly by. He dropped to his knees and began pressing down on Mr. Jones's chest, desperation guiding his hands. Another called 911, his voice urgent against the icy wind.

Minutes later, the paramedics arrived, taking over the relentless battle against death. Chest compressions, bag-mask ventilation, intubation, shocks from the defibrillator—their efforts were unyielding as they rushed Mr. Jones to the emergency room.

Inside the ER, the team sprang into action. Medications, ventilations, compressions—it was a whirlwind of calculated movements and clinical precision. The odds were against them, but they weren't ready to give up. Then, miraculously, after what felt like an eternity, a faint pulse returned. ROSC—Return of Spontaneous Circulation. The staff exchanged glances, knowing they had won the battle, but the war was far from over.

I was the assigned nurse that day. It was my job to meticulously manage the post-cardiac arrest care. Vasopressors to maintain blood pressure, anti-arrhythmic drugs to stabilize the heart, fluids, ventilator settings—every second was crucial as we prepared Mr. Jones for transfer to a larger hospital with specialized cardiac services.

As I worked, Mr. Jones's family arrived, their faces lined with worry and hope. They begged to see him, and recognizing the importance of their presence, I led them to his bedside. One by one, they whispered words of encouragement, telling him to get well, reminding him that he was loved. Among them stood Ezekiel, the man who had performed CPR on him. His expression was a mix of relief and lingering fear.

"Do you think he can hear me?" Ezekiel asked hesitantly.

I nodded at him. "I'm sure he can."

Leaning down, I began to speak softly into Mr. Jones's ear. "Mr. Jones, your family is here with you. Your daughter is by your side, and most importantly, the man who saved your life is standing right here, on your right."

A few seconds passed. Then, defying all odds, Mr. Jones's eyes fluttered open. Slowly, he turned his head to the right, his gaze settling on Ezekiel. A faint but unmistakable smile spread across his lips around the endotracheal tube. With great effort, his trembling right hand reached out—a silent but profound gesture of gratitude. Emotion swelled in the room, and tears welled in every eye.

Months later, while working in the ER, I was approached by one of my coworkers, Jeanne Emrick, who leaned in with a knowing smile. "You're not going to believe who just walked in," she said, gesturing toward a familiar face at the entrance. Mr. Jones had returned—not for a cardiac issue, but for a simple wound recheck. I walked over to him with my hand extended and he grabbed it, squeezing it with quiet strength.

“Thank you,” he said, his voice thick with emotion. “Thank you for not giving up on me.”

I smiled, watching the man who had once teetered on the edge of life and death now standing strong before me. Some days, the ER was filled with heartbreak, but on days like this, it was very much filled with miracles.

12 BALLS TO THE WALL

The ER was already a chaotic scene that morning, buzzing with the usual rhythm of sirens, hurried footsteps, and beeping monitors. But the moment the doors swung open, allowing the paramedics to wheel in a flailing, combative woman, the entire department seemed to tighten. She was thrashing, kicking, and screaming incoherent nonsense, her pupils blown wide, and sweat pouring from her face.

"She smoked that fake weed," one of the paramedics grunted, tightening his grip on the stretcher rail as the woman bucked wildly. "K2, Spice, whatever they're calling it these days. She's out of her mind."

Our ER staff had seen this before. Synthetic marijuana was a wildcard, triggering anything from seizures to psychosis. Today, it had turned this woman into a full-force hurricane of fists and feet. As soon as we moved her to a hospital bed, she lashed out, catching one of our nurses, Robert, on the arm and narrowly missing my face. She would have probably connected if my son, Cade Hall, an ER technician, hadn't put up his arm to block it. It took nearly six of us to wrestle her into four-point restraints, and even then, she fought like a caged animal.

Cade was a senior in high school and he worked with me in the ER on the weekend. Cade was used to handling difficult patients, but this one was testing everyone's limits. Dr. Adamcryk, the ER physician, ordered a CT scan to rule out any head trauma. We had administered sedatives, but the woman still had enough fight in her to make the transport a challenge. Cade, myself and two other members flanked the stretcher, guiding it toward radiology.

We were almost there when it happened.

As we were going through the final doorway toward radiology, Cade became pinned between the door frame and the right-side stretcher rail. In a movement so quick it seemed impossible, the patient wrenched one restrained hand through the side railing. Before anyone could react, she latched onto Cade's most vulnerable region—his groin.

The pain was instant, blinding. Cade's entire body locked up as an unbearable pressure clamped down on his most sensitive anatomy. His face turned a deep, unnatural shade of red, his mouth opening in silent agony. He couldn't even muster a scream; the pain stole the air from his lungs.

"Get her off! Get her off him!" ER nurse, Mixie Becker, shouted.

But she wouldn't let go. Her grip tightened, knuckles white with effort. Cade's legs buckled, his vision blurred, and for a brief moment, he said he thought he might actually pass out.

It took four of us to pry at her fingers, working desperately to peel them from Cade's groin. When they finally succeeded, he stumbled backward, gasping, hands on his knees. We all hovered around him, torn between sympathy and barely containing our laughter.

"You good, Cade?" I asked, trying—and failing—not to smirk.

He couldn't answer immediately, still recovering from the trauma. When he finally did, his voice was hoarse. "No. No, I am absolutely not good."

Even now, years later, Cade swears he can still feel it—the ghost of that iron grip. It's the kind of memory that never fades, no matter how hard you try.

13 REDNECK LANDING ZONE

The call came in just after sunset—a single-vehicle crash on a lonely stretch of Highway 27, deep in rural South Alabama. Lieutenant Sid Stevenson, along with the rest of the local EMS and fire crew, rolled up to find a battered sedan overturned in the thick brush, its frame twisted around a massive oak. The driver, a young man in his twenties, was slumped halfway out of the broken windshield, unrestrained and barely conscious. His breathing was labored, and blood traced down the side of his face, onto the hood of his car, and then dripping into the dirt.

Bystanders had already gathered—country boys in lifted four-wheel drive pickup trucks, their floodlights illuminating the wreckage. A few had climbed down into the wreck, trying to help, while others stood back, hands on their hips, murmuring in low voices.

Stevenson quickly assessed the scene. The driver was pinned—extrication was going to be a challenge. "We're going to need a helicopter," he muttered, pulling out his radio.

"Fire Dispatch, this is Lieutenant Sid Stevenson, requesting MAST for a trauma patient," he said, relaying coordinates. The dispatcher confirmed, and as soon as he ended the call, he turned back to his crew and the crowd.

"Alright, listen up!" he barked. "We need to clear out a place for the helicopter to land!"

A few of the country boys exchanged glances.

Satisfied that he had given the order, Sid returned to the vehicle to assist with extrication. The sound of hydraulic cutters filled the night air as his crew worked to free the driver. Then, over the controlled chaos, another sound cut through—something sharp, something mechanical.

"Chainsaws"

Stevenson's head snapped up. "What the hell?"

He turned, and to his disbelief, several of the country boys were deep in the woods, cutting down trees with chainsaws.

Lieutenant Stevenson stormed out, arms flailing about. "What in the hell are you guys doing?" he hollered over the roar of the saws.

One of them, a guy in a camo hat and a sleeveless flannel, looked up and grinned. "Clearing out a place for the helicopter to land, man!"

Stevenson just stared for a second, speechless. Then he exhaled sharply, shaking his head. "Y'all pack that crap up. Now."

Grumbling, the boys shut off their saws and started heading back to their trucks.

By the time the MAST chopper arrived, the fire crew had cleared a proper landing zone in a nearby field—one that didn't involve taking down half the forest. The patient was safely loaded up and flown out, his chances of survival much better thanks to the fast response.

As the chopper disappeared into the dark sky, Stevenson glanced back at the country boys leaning against their trucks, watching like it was the biggest show in town. He shook his head again, unable to stop a small grin.

"Only in South Alabama," he muttered, walking back to his rig.

Soon after, the UH1 MAST helicopter, along with the EMS crew and the patient, touched down at the local hospital.

Inside the ER, the trauma team had already assembled. The radio report had given them a few precious minutes to prepare: young male, unrestrained driver, prolonged extrication, head and chest trauma, possible internal injuries.

The trauma bay doors swung open as the flight crew and medics wheeled in the gurney. Blood spattered across the young man's torn shirt, dried in places, fresh in others. His right leg was visibly deformed—likely a femur fracture—and he had a jagged gash along his forehead, still oozing despite field dressing. His oxygen saturation was dropping, and his GCS hovered around 8. The ER nurses wasted no time.

"On my count—one, two, three—move!" said the lead nurse, Connie Johnstone, as they transferred him to the hospital stretcher. She was all business, her voice firm but calm.

Dr. Wayne Carlson, the attending ER physician that night, leaned over the patient and did a quick assessment.

"Get me vitals, stat. Two large-bore IVs, wide open with fluids. Type and crossmatch for at least 4 units. Let's get a portable chest and pelvis X-ray down here now."

The team sprang into action. One nurse worked the IVs, while another cut away the shredded clothing. A respiratory therapist was at the head of the bed, managing the airway and bagging the patient while RT prepared for potential intubation.

The cardiac monitor beeped steadily—heart rate 142, blood pressure 84/54. He was going into shock.

"Dr. Carlson, BP's crashing," Connie called out, squeezing in another liter of LR.

"He's bleeding somewhere," Dr. Carlson said aloud, more to himself than anyone else. "Get him to CT as soon as he's stable enough to move."

But they didn't wait. The bedside ultrasound—FAST exam—revealed fluid in the abdomen. Internal bleeding.

"He's got free fluid. Could be his spleen or liver. Let the OR know we've got a trauma case coming. He won't tolerate a delay," Carlson said, already donning sterile gloves.

But before surgery, he had to be intubated. As the patient began to gasp more irregularly, RT handed Dr. Carlson the laryngoscope.

"Let's tube him," he said. "Suction ready?"

"Ready."

Carlson got the tube in with no difficulty. A burst of mist fogged the tube.

"Good breath sounds, bilateral. Tube's secure," RT confirmed, connecting him to the ventilator.

Meanwhile, X-ray techs were snapping images at lightning speed. The chest film showed multiple rib fractures, a possible pneumothorax. Without missing a beat, Carlson inserted a chest tube on the left side. A rush of air and blood drained out—his lung had partially collapsed.

"Chest tube in. Let's get him packed for surgery," Dr. Carlson ordered.

Connie moved fast, printing out the latest lab results and taping them to the chart for the surgical team. "OR's ready," she called out, and the trauma team wheeled the patient out with the surgical nurse in the lead.

The chaos quieted as the stretcher disappeared down the hall. Connie stood still for a moment, catching her breath.

"That kid's lucky," Dr. Carlson said, pulling off his gloves and tossing them in the trash. "He should've died in that car."

Connie nodded slowly. "Or in the woods... if those country boys had cleared a little more 'landing zone.'"

They both cracked a tired smile.

Only in South Alabama.

And only in the ER.

14 Code Blue & Bedsheets

The double doors of the emergency department slammed open with the familiar chaos of a full arrest. The paramedics rushed in, compressions in progress, monitor wires trailing, and a bag-valve mask rhythmically hissing. The patient, a middle-aged male in his early 50s, was sprawled across the stretcher—unconscious, pulseless, and cyanotic. Sweat glistened on the brow of the lead medic as he called out:

"Fifty-three-year-old male, cardiac arrest. Found apneic and pulseless—VFib on initial rhythm. Defib twice, no ROSC. Down time approximately 10 minutes prior to our arrival. CPR in progress, epi x2 administered. ETA to ER was 4 minutes."

Behind the medics, chaos had another name: *the partner.*

A disheveled woman in her late 40s, wearing a bedsheet like a toga, stormed into the trauma bay behind them, screaming over the controlled urgency of the resuscitation team.

I *TOLD YOU* this would happen!" she bellowed, hands flailing as she stood in the middle of the ER waiting room, voice echoing off the walls. "He starts, but doesn't finish—*AGAIN!*" She pointed toward the triage doors like they were a courtroom exhibit. "You think I'm kidding? He just *STOPPED*—right in the middle—and rolled back like he was asleep. As if he *forgot* he was in the act! What kind of man—what kind of *grown man*—does that?"

Security was already moving in, ushering her to the family waiting room, but not before the ER charge nurse, Virginia Sampson, gave her a glance that said *you're not helping, ma'am.*

Dr. Tom Flowers, a seasoned ER doc with too many midnight shifts under his belt, barked out orders as his gloved hands intubated the patient.

"Get a line in him. Draw blood. Let's get a full panel including troponin, tox screen, and a type and cross—just in case. Charge the pads to 200. On my count—clear!"

The defibrillator gave a familiar whine. The body arched slightly with the shock.

"Still no pulse," said Virginia. "PEA now."

Dr. Flowers sighed, switching to his second pair of gloves. "Alright, let's work the Hs and Ts."

A nurse leaned in. "Medics said she was yelling about Viagra. Claims he 'popped two' about 30 minutes before arrest."

The doctor nodded grimly. "Alright—possible myocardial infarction or arrhythmia. Overdose? Maybe even a dissection. Someone get a history—*minus* the theatrics."

In the family room, the partner was still fuming. She paced in circles, ranting to whoever would listen.

"I lit candles. I played Luther. He said he was ready. Then BAM—he drops like a rock. I thought he was faking it, like he's done before when he's tired! I slapped him twice!"

A waiting patient raised an eyebrow. "You—slapped him?"

"I mean, LIGHTLY! I thought he was just being lazy. I didn't know he was dying!"

Meanwhile, back in trauma, the ultrasound probe swept across the man's chest. The heart was barely twitching—electrical activity with no mechanical output.

"Tamponade unlikely. No pericardial effusion. Lungs are clear—no pneumothorax. No signs of PE," the doctor called out.

After another round of epi, compressions, and defib, the monitor beeped with promise.

"Hold compressions!" Dr. Flowers leaned in.

"Sinus rhythm... wait—YES! We have a pulse!" Virginia called out.

The room collectively exhaled.

"Let's get him ready and up to the ICU. Notify cardiology. And someone please tell the girlfriend that screaming about unfinished business in the trauma bay, that it is not helping his myocardial recovery."

Later, as the ICU team took over and the ER reset for its next wave of chaos, Dr. Flowers looked up from his chart and muttered:

“Only in the ER can *performance issues* escalate into a full-blown code—one where coming and going at the same time becomes an actual medical reality.”

Virginia chuckled, sipping her coffee. “Can't make this stuff up.”

15 FULL MOON / GOLDEN SHOWER

It was Sunday night, and the full moon was out—high, bright, and clearly in charge of the madness flooding through the emergency department. The kind of night when you brace yourself for the absurd before even clocking in.

EMS rolled through the bay doors with a patient that looked like he'd been scraped off the underside of a house—which, as it turns out, was exactly where he'd been found.

"Male, approximately 40, found unresponsive under a raised home," the medic reported. "No obvious trauma, but he was totally unconscious, possibly intoxicated, so we immobilized him just to be safe."

The man was completely covered in dirt, twigs clinging to his hair, and his clothes damp with God-knows-what. They'd secured him in full spinal precautions: C-collar in place, chest and thigh straps tight across a backboard that still had flecks of gravel embedded in it. His skin was cold and clammy, and the scent coming off him was a potent mix of cheap liquor, soil, and poor decisions.

Me being the lucky one, stepped in to take report, eyebrows raised at the sight. The guy hadn't moved once since being wheeled in. I leaned over and gave him a hard sternal rub.

"Let's see if you're in there, buddy..."

The man groaned and stirred. His eyelids fluttered open, pupils sluggish, and he began mumbling. It was broken English—thick, slurred, barely intelligible. I caught fragments, but nothing coherent.

"Okay, alright, you're waking up," I said calmly. "Just hang tight, we're going to take *Bueno* care of you."

I turned around to grab the blood pressure machine when I heard the first call:

"Señor! Pee!"

I half-turned. "Okay, I'll get you a urinal—just one sec—"

"Señor... PEE! PEE PEE!!"

There was desperation now, a rising urgency in his voice that sounded like a man on the brink of disaster. Then, suddenly—

SSSSSSSS - CAWWWWK - GURGLE-GURGLE-GURGLE!

I quickly whipped around.

What I saw stopped me cold.

The man had somehow maneuvered a hand beneath the backboard immobilizer strap, unzipped his pants, and was now actively urinating—in his own face.

His head, still restricted by the C-collar, tilted back at just the right angle for the stream to hit him square between the eyes. It ricocheted off his nose and cheeks, running down into his ears, soaking his shirt, and baptizing the bed sheets in yellow. He jerked his head side to side in a futile attempt to dodge the spray, but the more he moved, the more chaotic the trajectory became.

It was a full-blown fountain of poor timing and even worse aim.

The urine hit the wall, the head of the stretcher, and part of the heart monitor. One of the straps slipped off his shoulder, exposing more skin to the cascade.

I stood there—urinal in hand, mouth slightly open, caught somewhere between complete utter amazement, disgust, and the kind of humor only an ER nurse could appreciate.

Another ER nurse, Shelley Whitehurst, walked by, paused, and peeked in.

"Oh my God… Jimmy, is he… peeing in his own face?"

I didn't look away. "Yep. And I'm just letting him finish. I mean, what do you even *do* with that?"

After the stream mercifully slowed and finally stopped, the man let out a relieved sigh, then mumbled something in Spanish—his tone peaceful, like a man who had conquered his mountain.

I stepped forward and hit the call light. "Yeah, uh… housekeeping to Room 18. We need a mop and possibly a hazmat suit."

I looked at the soaked mess before me, then muttered to myself: "A full moon never seems to disappoint."

And as the night rolled on and the next radio call buzzed through, I completed my charting and added a note:

"Pt found under house. Alert to voice. Initiated spontaneous urination with very poor aim and control."

16 DIY Urethral Stent

It was just after 8 pm when he came in—walking gingerly, legs slightly apart, one hand resting protectively over his groin like he was trying to hide something the whole world had already figured out. The triage nurse, Kimberly, gave him a quick once-over, her face unreadable. Years of ER madness had trained her to keep her reactions neutral, no matter what walked—or waddled—through the door.

"Name?"

"Uh… Chance."

"Last name?"

"Do I have to give it?"

"Yes."

A brief pause. "Lovett."

"Okay, Mr. Lovett," Kimberly said, typing into her computer. "What brings you to the ER tonight?"

He hesitated. Then he whispered it—so low she had to lean in. "There's a... straw. A fast-food straw. Super glued. Inside my..."

She blinked. "You said *super glued*?"

He nodded, red-faced. "Yes, ma'am."

She stared at him for a beat, then motioned for the tech to grab a room. "Right this way."

Room 12 was one of the small exam rooms, but it may as well have been a stadium the way Chance looked around nervously, as if the walls themselves might start laughing.

Dr. Bob Weaver was the ER physician that night—gruff, gray-bearded, and running on caffeine and sarcasm. He walked into the room with his usual dry wit.

"So, you decided to redecorate your urethra, huh?"

Chance sat up, clutching the thin hospital gown. "I just... it was a dare."

"Of course it was," Weaver replied, putting on gloves. "Nobody ever super glues a straw in their penis because it seemed like a good idea *on their own.*"

Carla Blackmon, ER nurse, gently pulled back Chance's gown while Weaver gently examined the area. Sure enough, there it was—a yellow-striped plastic burger joint drinking straw, with about 2 inches of it protruding from the tip of the penis. The remaining portion of the straw appeared to be embedded inside the urethra. Worse yet, the outer part of the penis was hardened with a thick ring of dried glue.

"It burns when I pee," Chance added, as if that somehow needed clarification.

"Yeah," Weaver said dryly, "that's called chemistry."

Urology was paged.

Dr. Mark Stone, the urologist on call, arrived about 45 minutes later—eye drops in, hair tousled, and no sign of excitement to be called in for what the nurse charted as "Foreign Body Insertion - Fast Food Straw."

He examined the situation, muttering under his breath, then gave the most anticlimactic answer of the night.

"Well," Stone said, removing his gloves and tossing them into the bin, "there's nothing I can do with that."

Chance's face fell. "What do you mean?"

"I mean," Stone said, folding his arms, "you super glued a straw into your urethra. It's adhered to the mucosa. I can't remove it without risking a full urethral tear. It's not obstructing flow, so the best thing to do... is wait."

"Wait?"

"Wait for the glue to wear off. Let nature work it loose. And pray you don't get a UTI or an infection in the meantime. Drink water. No... I take that back. Drink a *lot* of water. And no more arts and crafts with your junk."

Weaver, standing in the corner, smirked. "At least your urethra isn't obstructed. That's something."

Chance was discharged with strict instructions: fluids, antibiotics just in case, and an outpatient follow-up in a week. Carla handed him the discharge papers and a solemn warning: *If you feel like you're about to do something this stupid again… don't.*

As he left, one of the EMTs leaned over the counter. "Did that guy really have a straw—?"

"Yep," the Carla said, not missing a beat.

"In his—"

"Yep."

"Super glued?"

"Yep."

The EMT shook his head and whistled low. "And I thought I was having a rough night."

17 RUN! IT'S A MUDSLIDE!

It was a relatively calm afternoon in the emergency department—well, as calm as any ER ever gets. Chris Hovey, a seasoned ER nurse with nerves of steel and a stomach to match, was handling his assignment with the usual mix of efficiency and sarcasm.

One of his patients, an elderly gentleman with a weathered face and a stubborn streak, had been admitted for severe abdominal pain and obvious signs of constipation. After a bit of negotiation—and some blunt encouragement from the physician—Chris was given the noble task of administering a cleansing enema.

Chris, ever the professional, got everything prepped and proceeded with the procedure. The patient grumbled but cooperated. Within minutes, the enema did its job with almost *biblical* results. The patient leapt up, waddled urgently to the bedside commode, and let loose a catastrophic event that could be referred to as *The Brown Reckoning*.

Thinking the worst was over, the patient attempted to stand and move back to the stretcher. That's when disaster struck. His foot clipped the edge of the bedside commode—already weakened by the blast—and the entire toilet tipped over.

What came out was not a mere spill—it was a mudslide of epic proportions, cascading onto the ER floor in a steaming brown wave. The air instantly filled with a smell that could peel paint. Chris, now wide-eyed and frozen in disbelief, instinctively leapt back—only to realize there was nowhere safe to go.

Both he and the patient, now bonded through trauma, lunged onto the stretcher like it was a lifeboat escaping the Titanic. Chris barely made it, one foot dangling off the side as the flood reached beneath them. He slapped the nurse call button with a sense of desperation usually reserved for codes and cardiac arrests.

"Uh… I'm going to need some backup in here," he said over the intercom. "Major… overflow. Bring towels. Bring buckets. Bring a priest if one's available."

When his coworkers arrived, they found Chris perched on the stretcher like a stranded sailor, the patient beside him looking more embarrassed than ill, and the floor resembling a scene from a plumbing horror movie.

It took three nurses, two environmental services staff, and a healthy dose of humor to clean up the chaos. Chris eventually climbed down, soaked one shoe in bleach, and burned the other in the dumpster out back—just in case.

For weeks, he wouldn't walk past that room without side-eyeing the commode. And for months, whenever the ER staff heard a gurgle or felt a rumble in the floor, someone would whisper, "Remember the brown tsunami..."

And Chris would just nod, stare off into the distance, and say, "Some things you can't unsee."

18 A Can of Whoop Ass

It was a sticky summer evening in the 1980's, and the ER was just beginning to settle into the rhythm of the night shift. Back in those days, before the new hospital opened up across town, Steve Hartman, ER nurse recalls that they worked out of an old brick building with narrow halls, flickering fluorescent lights, and a constant hum of drama. The waiting room smelled faintly of cleaning solutions and your grandmother's old house, and the old air conditioning units did their best to keep up with the South Alabama heat.

Steve was restocking room supplies when a car pulled into the ambulance bay—not uncommon, since folks would often bypass the front entrance when they thought something was *real* serious. But this wasn't your usual chaotic arrival. The driver's door opened, and out stepped a neatly dressed African American woman in her early 40s—pressed blouse, slacks, earrings that swung just slightly as she walked.

She didn't run. She didn't yell. She just strolled into triage with the casualness of someone asking for a prescription refill.

Steve looked up from the nurses' station.

"Ma'am, can I help you?"

Without blinking, she said in the most matter-of-fact tone imaginable: "Yeah. I got my boy out in the car. I knocked him out."

That caught everyone in hearing distance in mid-step.

"You *what* now?" Steve asked, blinking.

"I knocked him out," she repeated, as if it were the most natural thing in the world. "He's in the backseat."

So out they went—to the old Buick parked in the bay.

Sure enough, slumped across the back seat was a teen boy, maybe 16 or 17. Semi-conscious, groaning softly, blood trickling down the side of his face. He had a C-shaped laceration just above his eyebrow, like something had caught him square in the forehead and folded the skin open like a flap on a cereal box. It wasn't deep enough for real alarm, but it definitely earned him a trip inside.

Steve got him in a wheelchair and brought him through the trauma room doors. He was groggy but responsive, no signs of a severe head trauma. Still, a head wound's a head wound, so they started working him up—neuro checks, vitals, and ordered an X-ray.

Meanwhile, his mama stood by the bedside, arms crossed, perfectly calm.

"Ma'am," one of the nurses asked, "can you tell us exactly what happened?"

She sighed and launched into her story, like she'd been waiting for someone to ask.

"Well, I was fixin' to go to the grocery store," she began. "And I could tell he'd been smoking that weed again. Eyes red, actin' all dumb. I got on his ass about it. Told him he better lay off that damn weed or he was going to fry what's left of his little brain."

She paused, adjusting her purse on her shoulder.

"So I went on to the store. Did my shopping, came home. I'm unloading groceries when he comes wandering in the kitchen, all red-eyed like he thinks I'm stupid. Still smellin' like that weed. I told him again—*'Boy, I know what you are doing' and I ain't having' it.'* That's when he got smart with me. Started mouthing off."

She shook her head and gave us the finale.

"I had a can of soup in my hand. Didn't even think about it. I just whipped it across the kitchen. Caught him right in the forehead. Knocked him out."

Steve tried to keep his face neutral. The ER physician, standing next to him, cleared his throat behind a smirk.

"Do you happen to recall what kind of soup it was?" Dr. Jones asked dryly.

"Cream of mushroom," she replied, without hesitation. "I was making casserole that night."

The boy, now a little more alert, winced as they cleaned the wound. Steve asked him if he remembered what happened. He blinked at them, then slowly turned his head to look at his mother, who was staring back at him with that look only Southern mamas can give—the kind that could melt asphalt.

"Yeah..." he muttered. "I remember now."

His X-ray came back clean. No skull fracture. Just a minor concussion and a forehead laceration that needed a few stitches, gave the usual discharge instructions, and sent him on his way.

As they walked out, he trailed behind her a few steps, head hung low, holding an ice pack to his forehead. She walked tall, calm, and victorious—like a general returning from battle. When they reached the car, she turned and said something low to him that Steve couldn't hear, but judging by the way he straightened up and snapped to the passenger seat, it was probably the end of *that* discussion.

They never saw him back in our ER again. No more weed-related soup-can incidents.

And to this day, whenever Steve hears someone say, "Spare the rod, spoil the child," he is quickly reminded of that woman……and that can of cream of mushroom soup.

19 HOT LESSON LEARNED

The smell hit first.

Burnt hair. Melted plastic. Gasoline. A pungent, acrid cocktail that clung to every corner of the emergency room like a ghost that refused to leave.

It was just past 6:00 PM on a muggy Tuesday evening when the double doors of the ER slammed open. A tall, broad-shouldered man in a soot-streaked T-shirt stormed in, cradling a limp teenage boy in his arms. The boy's skin was blotchy red and blistering, his face swollen, hair singed to his scalp. His arms looked like wax paper left too close to a flame. The man's voice cracked as he barked out, "Burns! Second, maybe third degree! I need help—now!"

He didn't have to say much more.

The nurses recognized the man instantly—Captain Jerry Thompson from station 1. Twenty-two years with the department. Decorated. Respected. A mentor to most of the rookies. But tonight, the fire wasn't something he ran toward. Tonight, the fire came for his only son.

The trauma team swept in fast. Monitors beeped as IVs were started, vitals checked, and saline dripped into cracked skin. A nurse gently cut away melted T-shirt fabric from the boy's chest while another hovered with pain meds, ready for the go-ahead.

The boy's name was Jackson—sixteen years old, six feet tall, and normally full of the kind of cocky teenage energy that made his mother both laugh and sigh. Now he just whimpered under his breath, eyes fluttering open long enough to catch the lights overhead before they rolled back again.

"What happened?" Dr. Andrews asked, glancing at Jerry.

Jerry wiped a trembling hand over his face, leaving behind a black streak of soot. "I—I don't know what the hell he was thinking. He ran out of gas. I was finishing a shift and came home to this… this madness."

A nurse paused. "He set himself on fire?"

Jerry exhaled hard, the words catching in his throat. "He tried to siphon gas from his truck in order to remove the gas tank for repair. But instead of using a hose, he grabbed a damn shop vac from the garage. He thought it'd be faster."

Everyone in the room froze for just a beat. The implications hit like a thunderclap. Shop vacs have electric motors. Electric motors produce sparks.

Gasoline vapors don't ask questions.

Jackson's burns were extensive—mostly second degree with some patches of first degree along his right forearm and jawline. His eyelashes were gone, his eyebrows too. Blisters were already ballooning along his upper chest and cheeks. The plastic tubing from the vacuum had literally fused to part of his shirt before it melted away.

"I taught him better," Jerry muttered later, standing outside the trauma bay with arms crossed tight over his chest. "He's watched me run fire safety drills. Seen the aftermath of careless mistakes. And still…"

Dr. Andrews placed a hand on his shoulder. "Kids don't think it'll happen to them. You know that. Doesn't matter if their dad's a fire captain or the president."

Jerry didn't answer, just stared through the glass at the pale figure of his boy—bandaged and quiet under warm lights. A different kind of burn settled behind the man's eyes—guilt.

Jackson was stabilized, pain managed, burns cleaned and dressed. The burn team was called in, and a plan was made to transfer him to the regional burn center. He'd heal, they said. Slowly, painfully—but he would heal.

Later that night, while prepping Jackson for transport, a nurse overheard him whisper through dry lips, "Did Dad tell y'all I blew the windows out of the garage?"

"No, honey," she said softly. "He didn't."

Jackson smiled faintly. "I thought I was being smart. Thought I'd go viral for fixing my truck with a vacuum. Now I'm going to look like Freddy Krueger."

Later that day, a young EMT stood outside the ER and watched as the helicopter lifted Jackson into the orange sky. Jerry stood beside him, silent. No uniform today—just a man, a dad, trying to make peace with the mistake he didn't make, but still somehow felt responsible for.

"He's going to be alright," the EMT offered.

Jerry nodded. "Yeah. He'll heal. But I'll never stop asking myself why I wasn't there to stop it."

The EMT paused, then said something simple.

"Maybe this'll be the story he tells that saves someone else."

As he reached for the door handle on his truck, Jerry blinked and looked out toward the clouds, a tear finally breaking free. "God, I hope so."

20 Final Words from a Hero

ER nurse, Zack Marden recalls a story when he was barely eighteen years old—fresh out of high school, green as spring grass, and proudly wearing his navy blue hospital scrubs. Being a new ER tech, he was eager to do anything, everything. Stocking linen, pushing wheelchairs, mopping floors—whatever they needed him to do, he was there with wide eyes and willing hands. But what he loved most, what filled something deep in his chest, was the chance to slow down and talk to patients. Especially the old timers.

Back then, the ER wasn't quite the nonstop war zone it is today. They had moments—brief, golden moments—when things were quiet. And in those moments, Zack would drift toward the rooms where the elderly patients sat alone, eyes half-closed under the hum of the recognizable ER operating sounds, often just waiting. Waiting for tests. Waiting for discharge. Waiting for... something.

It was a quiet Sunday afternoon when Zack walked into one of those rooms. A small room, lights low, with the soft rhythmic beep of the heart monitor keeping time like a metronome. In the bed lay an older gentleman—easily in his eighties. His arms were thin, but his hands were massive, calloused, with veins that looked like rivers running beneath weathered skin.

"Hey there, sir," Zack said gently. "Can I get you anything?"

The man turned his head slowly and blinked up at him. "Yeah," he said in a gruff voice. "Who do I report to?"

It caught Zack off guard. "Excuse me?" he said.

He shifted slightly, looking irritated. "I said—who's in charge? I need to speak to the officer."

Zack blinked, unsure. "Uh… I guess that would be the charge nurse. But she's a… well, she's a she."

He let out a disappointed grunt. "The Army's gone to hell," he muttered. "Alright, fine. Let me see her then."

Zack smiled. "She's tied up right now, but I'll let her know."

He gave a begrudging nod, then squinted at him. "What outfit you with?"

That's when it started to click.

"Oh—I don't know." Zack said with a small laugh. "I just work here, sir."

He scoffed. "Orderly, huh? Damn shame. Strapping boy like you ought to be carrying shells. Back in my day, I could haul a 105 on each shoulder, up and down the line all damn day."

He laid his head back, and his eyes softened. Zack pulled up a chair beside him.

For the next hour, he took Zack back in time.

He told him about the beaches in Normandy—how the sand was red by the time he hit it. About the cold of Korea—how it bit at your bones worse than any bullet. About buddies who never made it home, and the quiet that followed after the firefights. His voice would rise and fall like he was back there, every word painting vivid pictures. Zack just sat there, hanging on every one of them.

Eventually, a call came in, and Zack had to run something upstairs. He stood to leave.

"Well, sir, I've got to go, but I'll be back to check on you." Zack said.

He nodded slowly. "That's fine. I'm tired anyway. Might close my eyes for a bit."

"Thank you for the stories." Zack told him.

He gave a faint smile and closed his eyes.

Zack left the room.

An hour or so later, he came back downstairs and glanced at the patient board. A thin red line ran across his name.

We all knew what that meant.

"Hey... what happened to Mr. Berkshire?" Zack asked a nurse quietly.

She glanced up from her charting. "He was a DNR. Brady'd down in his sleep. Peaceful."

Zack just stood there, stunned. He had *just* talked to him. He had been there. Real. Alive. Telling stories.

Zack felt a weird tightness in his chest. It wasn't the first time he'd seen death. But this was the first time it had spoken to him an hour before.

Not long after, a man walked up to the nurses' station—mid-fifties, baseball cap in hand, eyes red-rimmed but steady.

"Hey," he said, looking around. "I'm Mr. Berkshire's son, Tim. Someone told me you were the last person to talk to my dad?"

Zack stood up and said, "Yes sir, I sat with him for about an hour. He told me some great stories."

The man stepped in a little closer, his voice low and tentative. "Can I ask what he said? I mean… if you remember. Everything?"

Zack nodded. It was still fresh, playing in his mind like a movie on loop. So Zack told him. Every story. Every detail that he could remember. Normandy. Korea. The artillery shells. The cold. The silence.

Tim Berkshire didn't interrupt. Just stood there, absorbing it all. His eyes shimmered. When Zack finished, he stepped forward, grabbed Zack's hand in both of his, and then pulled him into a hug.

"Thank you," he whispered. "You don't know what that means. Dad never talked about his time in the war. Not even after I enlisted. I always wanted to know. I guess he finally had to get it off his chest. And… thank God you were here."

He stepped back, wiped his eyes, and smiled.

"God bless you, son."

And just like that, he turned and walked away.

Zack stood there, stunned and honored. He didn't know what to say.

But he will tell you this—He *never forgot that old man.*

And to this day, no matter how slammed the ER is, no matter how long the to-do list is, he always makes time for the old timers. Especially the veterans.

Zack said proudly, "Because you never know when they just might need to talk…

…or when you might be the last person to hear them."

21 CATCHING A BUZZ

It was just after 9 a.m. when the calm rhythm of a new-day lull was shattered by the sudden blare of shouting echoing through the ambulance bay.

A female police officer—uniform rumpled, eyes wide with panic—burst through the double doors like a freight train of desperation. Her right hand pounded the side of her head, her movements wild and erratic.

"GET IT OUT! GET IT OUT!" she screamed, shaking her head violently. Her voice cracked with agony, each syllable a raw plea. She wasn't just panicked—she was in excruciating pain, and something about her frantic, repetitive motion set the whole department on high alert.

Blood pressure monitors were silenced. Patients in nearby bays turned their heads. Nurses froze mid-chart. The officer staggered forward, gasping through gritted teeth, still hitting the side of her head with the heel of her hand like she was trying to beat something out of her skull.

Dr. Drew Johns was the first to react. A former Navy combat medic turned ER physician, Drew had seen all kinds of chaos, but this—this was different. With swift precision, he moved toward her, his voice calm but firm.

"Ma'am, come with me—now."

She offered no resistance, her trust in the badge-to-badge bond shining through her terror. He guided her into ER Bay 5, motioning for a nurse to close the door behind them. As she sat on the stretcher, still writhing and yelping in pain, she managed to blurt out between gasps:

"I was on a traffic stop—on the side of Highway 84—when something *flew* into my ear. A bug. I tried to get it out. I did. But it just—*it went in deeper!* It's in there, it's buzzing—buzzing like a chainsaw!"

Dr. Johns nodded with understanding. He gently guided her to lay down, turning her head so her right ear faced upward. Then, he did something unusual.

"Kill the lights," he ordered.

The overhead fluorescents blinked off. The room was suddenly dim, except for the small stream of orange light sneaking through the edge of the door. Then, he flicked on the overhead surgical lamp—a high-intensity beam—and slowly positioned it a few inches above the officer's ear canal.

"Hold still," he whispered. "Don't move. Just trust me."

Everyone in the room stood still, watching with silent curiosity. The room was so quiet that you could hear the air conditioner hum.

And then—like something out of a science fiction movie—it happened.

A small slender black insect *launched* from her ear canal, flitting in circles before zipping off toward the door and disappearing. The officer let out a sharp gasp, then collapsed onto the stretcher with a long, ragged sigh. Relief washed over her face like a wave crashing over hot pavement after a summer storm.

The room remained in stunned silence for a few seconds.

"...What the hell just happened?" murmured an ER tech, Joseph.

Dr. Johns smirked slightly. "The bug flew into her ear—a dark tunnel. Turn off the lights, shine a bright light at the exit, and let nature find its way out."

"That's it?" ER nurse Liz asked, blinking. "That simple?"

"That effective," he replied, peeling off his gloves.

The officer, still catching her breath, sat up slowly. "I'd take getting tased over that *any* day," she muttered.

Someone chuckled, and the tension in the room finally broke. A slow round of applause echoed among the staff, not for dramatics—but out of genuine awe.

They had all witnessed something rare: an elegant, non-invasive medical trick that required no instruments, no trauma, no meds—just understanding of the way the world works and a well-aimed light.

As the officer stood and straightened her duty belt, she gave a sheepish salute.

"Thanks, Doc," she said, her voice husky. "I owe you."

Dr. Johns just grinned. "Next time you pull someone over, maybe wear earplugs."

The officer laughed—truly laughed—and walked out of Bay 5 a new woman. The staff, still marveling at the simplicity of the solution, added the incident to their growing mental catalog of unbelievable ER stories.

And somewhere out there, a very confused bug was likely questioning its life choices.

22 SEE SPIDER—RUN!

The emergency department had seen its fair share of chaos over the years—traumas, code blues, combative psych patients, and the occasional patient attacked by the ferocious South Alabama Bush Hog. But if there was one thing that brought a sense of levity and laughter to the staff in the midst of it all, it was ER nurse Terry Olive.

Terry was more than just a seasoned nurse—he was the unofficial morale officer of the hospital. With a quick wit, a heart of gold, and a love for mischief, Terry made it his mission to bring a little joy into the sterile walls of the ER. And while he decorated for every major holiday—Valentine's hearts in triage, shamrocks dangling from the IV poles in March, and a full-blown Fourth of July flag wall behind the nurses' station—there was one holiday that he took far more seriously than the rest: Halloween.

For Terry, Halloween wasn't just a holiday—it was *his* holiday.

Every year, he began planning weeks in advance. He'd sketch out haunted house blueprints in the break room, take polls on what horror theme to go with, and spend his off days at dollar stores and craft shops, collecting skeletons, cobwebs, and animatronic bats. The ER turned into something between a trauma bay and a movie film set by mid-October. But nothing ever topped the year of *The Spider Incident.*

That particular October, Terry's creative spark was ignited by a clearance rack at a hardware store. There, in a dusty bin, he found an oversized black Halloween spider—plastic legs outstretched, red beady eyes, and a body the size of a football. Inspiration struck immediately.

What if the spider could drop down on visitors as they entered the ER?

Now, Terry wasn't just a nurse—he was also a tinkerer. But this time, he was aiming big.

He spent days rigging the spider with a pulley system, attaching fishing line to the automatic ER bay doors—the very ones ambulances backed up to and walk-ins often entered through. The idea was simple: when the outer doors opened, the movement would trigger the spider to slowly descend from the overhead awning just outside, giving the illusion of a massive arachnid dropping from the sky.

Terry tested it—over and over. He added weight to the spider for smoother descent, adjusted the drop angle, and even programmed a slight "bounce" at the bottom, just to add to the realism. Staff members were invited to preview the effect. Some laughed, others yelped, and one hospital orderly nearly dropped his coffee. Terry took that as a win.

Then came *the day*.

It was a calm afternoon. A low hum of activity buzzed in the background of the ER. Patients were being triaged, vital signs charted, nurses doing what they always did—balancing compassion, urgency, and caffeine.

Terry had just finished rechecking the spider rig one last time, satisfied with the slow, deliberate drop it would perform when the sensor was triggered. He retreated back inside, grinning as he peeked through the glass, waiting for his next "test subject."

Then it happened. A middle-aged, well-dressed woman carrying a small purse, wearing walking shoes entered the perimeter outside of the bay doors. She didn't appear injured, wasn't in a hurry, just casually approaching the ER entrance from the parking lot. She was perhaps coming for chest pain. Or maybe to check on a family member. She might've had an urgent care-worthy rash or a headache that had lingered a little too long.

We'll never know.

Because just as she stepped within range of the automatic doors, the sensor fired. The outer glass panels whooshed open with their familiar hydraulic motion—and from the overhang above, the massive black spider descended.

Slowly.

Intentionally.

Right. Toward. Her. Head.

What happened next was witnessed by Terry and another ER nurse.

The woman froze—just for a second. Her eyes locked on the descending horror from the sky. Then, in a blur of pure survival instinct, she turned on her heel and bolted down the sidewalk with the kind of speed that would've made Olympic sprinters proud. She didn't pause, didn't scream, and didn't even glance back.

She just ran.

Out of the parking lot.

Past the corner of the neighboring building

Gone.

Terry and the nurse quickly decided that they should probably go see if they could stop her, but she was gone. Like she had just disappeared into thin air.

To this day, nobody knows who she was or why she was coming to the ER.

The story of Terry's Halloween spider became ER folklore. Told to new hires every fall. Shared at holiday parties and retold with increasing exaggeration year after year.

Terry Olive kept decorating every year, but perhaps toned it down just a bit. The spider, however, remained his proudest invention—even if it scared one woman clean out of the county.

In the wild world of emergency medicine, laughter and lightness were often rare commodities. And thanks to Terry, Halloween would always bring both.

Whether you were ready for it or not.

Terry Olive was an ER nurse whose legacy extended far beyond the walls of the emergency department. Known for his unwavering kindness and heartfelt compassion, Terry had a gift for making patients feel seen, heard, and valued—even in the most chaotic and frightening moments of their lives. His calming presence and gentle demeanor could bring peace to the most anxious of patients, and his quick wit often brought a smile to faces when it was needed most.

Among his coworkers, Terry was more than just a nurse—he was a friend, a mentor, and a light in even the darkest shifts. He never hesitated to lend a helping hand, offer a word of encouragement, or stay late to support a teammate in need. His infectious laughter and creative spirit—especially evident during his famously elaborate holiday decorations—brought life and joy to a place often burdened by pain and uncertainty.

Terry's care extended beyond clinical skill; it was rooted in genuine humanity. He believed that every patient deserved dignity, no matter their circumstances. Whether he was holding the hand of a frightened child, sitting quietly with a grieving family, or cracking a joke to ease the tension in a trauma room, Terry made a lasting impact on everyone he encountered.

Though he is no longer with us, Terry Olive's legacy lives on in the stories shared by those who knew him and in the hearts of the many lives he touched. His life was a testament to what it means to truly care—and to do so with consistency, humility, and grace.

23 CURTAIN CALL CATASTROPHE

It was just after 4 p.m. when rural EMS rolled in, lights off but siren still echoing in the minds of ER nurses Shelley Mae and Hazel Ray. They exchanged a glance. They already knew who it was.

"Frequent flyer inbound," Hazel Ray muttered, as she popped a piece of gum and pulled on a fresh pair of gloves.

Shelley Mae sighed. “Let me guess. Odorous, overdressed, and under-bathed?”

Bingo.

The patient, Ginny Mae Higginbotham—an older semi-homeless woman from the outskirts of the county, known for her chronic complaints and a scent that could wilt the strongest stomach—was wheeled in on the stretcher. Her hair was matted, her clothes stained and layered, and her scent? A potent mix of old sweat, cigarette smoke, and spoiled milk.

Shelley Mae and Hazel Ray were no rookies. Between the two of them, they had over 40 years of ER experience. They'd seen it all—until today.

They escorted her to a curtained room in the back corner of the ER, partly out of privacy, partly to protect the other patients from what was to come.

"Let's get you into a gown," Shelley Mae said with the kind of forced cheer that nurses reserve for when the situation is about to go sideways.

Ginny Mae groaned as they began peeling off layers of crusted clothing. The air grew heavier with each removed article. As Hazel Ray carefully untangled a pair of three-day-old leggings from her legs, Ginny Mae suddenly announced:

"I gotta go. Now."

Shelley Mae, quick to react, grabbed a bedpan from the cabinet and brought it bedside.

"Here, just use this. We'll help you—"

Before she could finish, she snatched the bedpan from Shelley's hands with surprising agility and squatted—naked, knees shaking, body trembling.

Then it happened.

A sound erupted that neither nurse would ever forget—like a water balloon filled with hot gravy being popped under pressure.

A violent, liquefied explosion.

The diarrhea hit the center of the bedpan with such force it deflected like a geyser, spraying horizontally in a perfect arc of destruction. It splattered the curtain, the bedframe, and the bottom of Hazel Ray's scrubs.

She screamed as Shelley Mae dove to the side like a soldier in a foxhole.

"Sweet Jesus, it ricocheted!" Hazel Ray shouted, wiping the bed rail with a towel that would immediately be sent to incineration.

The room filled with the unmistakable smell of gastrointestinal horror.

Just then—without warning—Dr. Hope pulled back the curtain with the poise of a man ready to diagnose a cough.

He stopped cold.

There, perched like a gargoyle on the rim of a steaming bedpan, was Ginny Mae. Naked. Victorious. Unapologetic.

The room was dripping. Literally. The curtain was streaked in brown sludge. The bed was stained like a war zone. The floor had trails.

Dr. Hope blinked once. Then twice. His nose twitched.

He slowly let the curtain fall back into place like a disappointed magician ending a failed trick.

"I'll... come back," he said quietly, already halfway down the hall.

Shelley Mae and Hazel Ray just stared at each other.

Hazel Ray broke the silence. "We need a priest."

"No," Shelley whispered. "We need a pressure washer."

And thus, "Curtain Call Catastrophe" became legend in the ER for years to come—retold with horror, humor, and a firm reminder: always approach a bedpan with caution... and never underestimate trajectory.

24 My Patient is—Dead!

The night shift in the ER had been relatively calm—until around 11:30 p.m., when EMS rolled in with an elderly man who had fallen at home. He was alert, in a lot of pain, and couldn't move his right leg. His name was Mr. Arthur Jennings, age 84, and he had what everyone suspected was a fractured hip.

With only two trauma bays in the ER, space was limited. But the charge nurse, Meghan Cole, was always thinking three steps ahead. They placed Mr. Jennings in Trauma Bay 1, started IV fluids, gave him pain control, and ordered X-rays, which confirmed the obvious: a clean intertrochanteric femur fracture. He would need surgery—just not tonight. The orthopedic surgeon wasn't available until early the following morning, so Mr. Jennings would have to wait in the trauma bay until the orthopedic team rounded.

Meanwhile, Trauma Bay 2 held a very different kind of patient.

Earlier that evening, a code had come in—a man in his 60s, cardiac arrest with no known history.

EMS worked him enroute, and the ER team took over for a grueling 45-minute code. Despite everyone's best efforts, the patient never regained a pulse. After the time of death was called, Meghan and another nurse stayed behind to clean the body, dress the man in a hospital gown, and place a clean sheet up to his chest. They dimmed the lights and set the room up so the family—who had just arrived—could say goodbye.

Afterward, the man's body remained in Trauma Bay 2, awaiting pickup from the local funeral home scheduled for early the next morning.

By 5:30 a.m., the unit was quiet again, bathed in the faint blue hue of monitors and hallway lights. Meghan, tired but efficient, prepped the paperwork for both patients—Mr. Jennings in Bay 1 for ortho surgery, and the deceased man in Bay 2 for the funeral home. She printed off face sheets, double-checked forms, signed what needed signing, and placed everything neatly into their respective chart binders.

Or so she thought.

At 6:03 a.m., Dr. Brady Fleming, the orthopedic surgeon, strode into the department with his usual pre-coffee frown and demanded the chart for the hip fracture. Meghan handed him Mr. Jennings's binder from the counter.

Without a word, he turned and entered the room.

Not thirty seconds later, he returned—pale, confused, and borderline panicked.

"My patient is dead!" he barked.

Meghan froze for a second, trying to process what he had just said.

"What?" she said.

"I just examined him. He's cold. He's *dead*! You handed me the chart—Trauma Bay 2, right?"

That's when it hit her. Her heart dropped to her stomach.

She lunged for the second chart on the counter and flipped it open. Sure enough, the funeral home paperwork—body release forms, time of death, death certificate copies—all neatly filed in the chart for Trauma Bay 1.

"Oh my God," she muttered. "Doc, I gave you the wrong chart."

Dr. Fleming blinked. "So... he's not dead?"

"No, sir. Your patient is in Bay 1. The dead one is in Bay 2."

He narrowed his eyes. "You're sure?"

"I promise. Jennings is very much alive. He's just old and not thrilled about the wait."

With a grunt, Dr. Fleming turned on his heel and marched into Bay 1—this time, to find a very living Mr. Jennings complaining about how long he had been waiting.

Back at the nurses' station, Meghan placed the two charts side by side and marked them both with bold labels: **ALIVE** and **DECEASED**—just to avoid another early morning resurrection.

25 SOGGY SITUATION

It was a slow mid-afternoon in the ER—a rare lull between the chaos. The kind of shift where boredom breeds bad decisions and prank wars bubble just below the surface.

Jake and Marcus, two seasoned ER nurses with a long-standing reputation for mischief, were manning the station. Jake was the brains of the operation, always scheming some harmless gag. Marcus? He was the executioner—the guy who couldn't keep a straight face even if he tried. Together, they were trouble. But the kind of trouble that made a long 12-hour shift bearable.

Jake was leaning back in his rolling chair, chewing the end of a pen. "You know that old cloth chair by the printer?" he said, eyes twinkling.

Marcus raised an eyebrow. "The one that sags like a wet diaper? What about it?"

"I think it's due for a hydration boost," Jake grinned, pulling a 60 mL syringe from his pocket.

Marcus laughed. "Saline?"

Jake nodded. "Let's give it a little… cushion surprise."

They ducked over to the chair like two teenagers with a water balloon. Jake knelt beside it and found a weak spot in the fabric where the threads were already worn. Carefully, he slipped the syringe tip beneath and began injecting saline into the foam cushion. It soaked up the fluid quietly, darkening slightly, but not enough to notice unless someone was really paying attention.

"Couple hundred milliliters should do it," Jake whispered like a surgeon working on a stealth operation. "Enough to feel wet… not enough to puddle."

Marcus gave a low whistle. "Who do you think will sit in it?"

Jake smirked. "Could be anyone. But I'm hoping for Sheila. She always acts like she's too good for this place."

They went back to work, casting sideways glances toward the chair every time someone wandered near it. Hours passed. A few near misses. A tech almost sat down but was called away at the last second. A nursing student hovered nearby but opted for a rolling stool instead. The anticipation was killing them.

And then, right around 4:15 p.m., it happened.

Dr. Alan Ford, the cardiologist, entered through the double doors with his usual swagger. Mid-50s, navy scrubs with a white coat crisply pressed, and a stethoscope that probably cost more than Jake's car. He was all business—buttoned-up, fast-talking, with the bedside charm of a toaster oven. He walked straight to the nurse's station, flipping through a clipboard.

Jake and Marcus locked eyes.

Dr. Ford set his folder down and, without a second thought, lowered himself onto *the chair*.

At first, there was silence. Then… a squish.

He paused.

His face twitched.

And slowly, very slowly, he stood up again.

Everyone nearby turned their heads in unison, watching as Dr. Ford examined the back of his pants. A large, dark, wet patch spread across the seat of his scrubs like a crime scene.

"What the hell is this?" he snapped, twisting to look at the chair, then back at the nurses.

Jake bit the inside of his cheek. Marcus had already ducked behind the workstation, shoulders shaking.

"Did someone spill something?" Dr. Ford demanded.

No one answered.

He stormed off down the hall, barking something about "changing clothes" and "unprofessionalism" and "how can you expect anyone to take this place seriously when it smells like a dog bowl and the chairs are soaked like a sponge?"

The door slammed behind him.

Jake waited until the coast was clear, then turned to Marcus. "Well," he said, "it wasn't Sheila."

Marcus wheezed with laughter. "We just gave the head of cardiology a wet butt. We're dead."

Later that week, an all-staff email came down from administration: *"Tampering with hospital furniture is grounds for disciplinary action."* The chair mysteriously disappeared the next day, replaced with a new plastic one—wipeable and waterproof.

Jake and Marcus never admitted to the prank, but the legend of the "Soaked Seat Incident" lived on. And for months afterward, every time Dr. Ford entered the nurse's station, he glanced twice before sitting—forever wary of hydrated cushions and mischievous nurses with syringes full of saline.

26 THE SOUND OF RETALIATION

For a very long time, I had been plotting a revenge prank on one of my emergency department coworkers. Mixie Becker, the undisputed queen of great pranks in the emergency department, had pulled off some legendary stunts, and now it was time for just a little payback. I had spent hours perfecting this plan, and today was the day it would all unfold.

The ER was already beginning to ramp up with the usual early-morning chaos of minor medical complaints when I began setting the stage. I made my rounds, stocking my rooms as usual, while discreetly placing my little secret weapon—a remote-controlled fart machine—inside a cabinet drawer directly behind the triage nurse's station desk. I wrapped the device inside of a bath towel to enhance its performance. The device had an impressive array of sounds, from mild to catastrophic pre-recorded explosions, and my plan was, well.... to use them all.

Earlier, right after shift change, I discreetly gathered the rest of the staff, giving them the rundown on my plan. The goal was simple: prank

Mixie in front of a patient in a way that she'd never see coming. The anticipation was electric as everyone took their positions, trying to maintain their composure.

Right on cue, Mixie escorted an elderly female patient into the triage room. As always, Mixie stood at the desk, with her back perfectly aligned and resting on the drawer, completely unaware of what was about to happen. I gripped the remote, waiting for the perfect moment. Then—pressing the button—I let the first one rip.

The muffled yet unmistakable sound of flatulence filled the small room. The patient's eyes widened slightly, but she remained composed, continuing to describe her symptoms in great detail to her triage nurse. Mixie, ever the professional, stiffened slightly but didn't react.

It wasn't over yet.

I pressed the button again. This time, the machine unleashed a thunderous, wet-sounding explosion. The nurses at the desk were barely holding it together, shoulders shaking as they suppressed their laughter. Mixie shot a death glare toward the nurse's station desk and mouthed the words "I'm going to kill you!", but I donned my prankster poker-face and remained the picture of innocence.

Then, for the grand finale, I hit the button once more. This time, the device let out an obnoxiously long, drawn-out, wet, "sheet ripping" fart! The sheer volume and duration of it sent the entire nurses' station into silent convulsions of laughter. One nurse actually had to turn away, tears streaming down her face.

Mixie's face turned a shade of red that would make a stop sign jealous. The patient, now eyeing Mixie with concern along with a sincere look that seemed to say, "Are you okay, sweetheart?"

That was it. The dam broke. The nurses at the station collapsed into full-blown, uncontrollable laughter. Even the charge nurse had to step away to keep from completely losing her composure. Mixie, mortified, clenched her jaw and shot daggers my way, while I continued to play the innocent bystander.

She had been punked. And not many people could say they had pulled one over on Queen Mixie. But I sure did!

From that day on, I knew that I had to keep my head on a swivel and my radar on. Retaliation was inevitable. My days were numbered. We all knew that Mixie was already plotting her revenge on me. But for now, I was marinating in the glory of a perfectly executed prank.

27 RUB LADY, RUB!

Some shifts start slow. Others come at you like a freight train. This one started somewhere in between—quiet enough to let your guard down, but with that uneasy lull that ER folks know means something's brewing. And sure enough, the call came in: Altered Mental Status, possible danger to self or others.

Translation? Buckle up.

Zack Marden, ER Nurse, recalls that EMS rolled in with a man in his early 30s—African American, about 6'4", and built like the side of a battleship. You ever see someone so jacked you feel like apologizing for your own existence? That was this guy. He looked like Apollo Creed after a steroid bender. Every muscle had muscles. Arms like tree trunks. Chest you could bounce quarters off of.

But here's the thing—he wasn't doing anything threatening. In fact, he was still. Real still. He sat upright on the stretcher, staring into some invisible void beyond the ambulance bay doors. His responses were clipped. "Yes." "No." "Fine." But his silence wasn't relaxed. It was *coiled.*

Trailing behind him was his wife. Barely five feet tall, very cute and petite, and every bit as calm as her husband. She followed close behind, concern etched across her face. She wasn't new to this. You could tell she'd been here before.

Turns out, he was a veteran—combat tours, PTSD, the whole nine yards. What made this one different, though, was the small electronic device he had surgically implanted in his chest: a vagal nerve stimulator.

None of us had seen one in use before.

"It's supposed to help when he starts to spiral," his wife explained softly. "I just rub the handheld device over his chest, right here—" she motioned with practiced ease, "—and it helps calm him down."

"Like a reset button?" Kimbo, our tech, asked.

"Exactly. But lately... it hasn't been working as well."

Alan nodded, he was assigned as the primary nurse, and he got to work doing his assessment. Zack stepped out of the room to catch up on charting, and Kimbo lingered behind to help Alan.

Everything seemed calm.

Until it wasn't.

Suddenly, Kimbo burst out of the room like her shoes were on fire. "ZACK!" she yelled. And let me tell you—when a tech calls your name like that, you *move.*

"I sprinted to the room and froze at the door", said Zack.

There was Alan—clinging like a toddler on a carnival ride—on the back of our now very *not calm* patient, who was walking slowly but with purpose right toward him. His eyes weren't on Zack, though. He was looking *through* him. Sweating. Breathing heavy. Whispering something about "getting his buddies." His mind wasn't in this room anymore.

It was back in the desert. Or on a convoy. Or in some flashback we couldn't understand.

"Where's the wife?!" Zack asked Kimbo, who was pressed against the wall in full "I don't get paid enough for this" mode.

"She ran out to the car! To get the stimulator!" Kim said.

So here they were. Alan trying to slow down this human freight train by riding him piggyback. Zack standing in front of him like he might actually stop him, even though he knew that the man could snap him like a pretzel. And Kimbo hovering behind Zack, whispering, "Oh crap, oh crap, oh crap."

Just when Zack was considering sacrificing Alan as a distraction, the wife burst back through the doors, holding the device like she was about to defuse a bomb.

She looked up at them and shouted, "WHAT DO YOU WANT ME TO DO?!"

Alan, still on the guy's back, didn't hesitate to yell.....

"**RUB, LADY! RUB!!**"

And she did.

She darted up to him, placed the device firmly over his chest, and began to rub in fast, practiced circles. At first—nothing. He kept muttering. Kept walking.

Then—like a flicker of light behind his eyes—he slowed. His muscles unclenched. His breathing eased. And then he stopped.

Alan slid down his back like a firefighter down a pole.

The man looked around, blinking like he'd just woken up from a dream. "Where am I?" he asked, confused but calm.

The team got him settled again, gave him a mild sedative for good measure, and made sure psych and the VA liaison were in the loop. His wife never left his side, her tiny hand resting on his arm the whole time. She was his anchor.

And Alan?

He had rug burns on his inner thighs from riding that man's back like a mechanical bull.

Later that night, back at the nurses' station, Zack, Alan, and Kimbo couldn't stop laughing. Every time they would get serious, Alan would suddenly bellow, "**RUB, LADY! RUB!**" and they'd fall out all over again.

But beneath the laughter was a deep respect—for the patient, for his story, and for the tiny woman who stood between the man she loved and the war still waging in his mind.

It was a wild night in the ER. One they would never forget.

And from then on, anytime something went sideways, you might hear the unofficial code phrase:

"Rub, lady... RUB!"

28 OF RICE & MEN

Early in my career, I had the privilege of working alongside Chuck Crawford, a fellow paramedic, when we both landed full-time positions in the emergency department of a local hospital. At the time, transitioning from the back of an ambulance to the fast-paced environment of the ER felt like stepping into an entirely new world. We were young, eager, and ready to take on the chaos that came through those double doors each day. Working in the ER gave us a front-row seat to both the raw intensity and quiet triumphs of emergency medicine—and having a trusted partner like Chuck by my side made those early years not only more manageable, but often unforgettable.

It was midmorning in the ER, the usual steady rhythmic sound of activity echoing through the halls—monitors beeping, phones ringing, and the occasional overhead page breaking through the white noise. I had just finished charting on a patient when the call light on the wall phone flashed. On the other end was Dr. Moorehouse, the orthopedic surgeon on call.

His voice was calm but direct, "You've got a patient coming in from a small rural hospital in Florida. Elderly female, post-op tib-fib fracture. Sounds like she's had a setback."

He went on to explain that the woman had recently undergone surgery for an open tibia and fibula fracture, and now—just weeks later—she had apparently fallen and re-injured the same leg. The referring hospital didn't have the resources to manage the complication, so they were transferring her to us for evaluation and further care. Dr. Moorehouse instructed me to remove her cast upon arrival and send her straight to radiology for updated X-rays. He'd be by later to examine her himself.

At the time, it sounded routine. Just another transfer, another post-op complication.

No problem, right?

The patient rolled in not long after, brought in by EMS and transferred gently onto our stretcher. She was an elderly woman with a kind face and the most pleasant Southern accent you could imagine. The kind of patient who made you want to slow down, smile, and listen to her tell stories about her garden, even in an emergency room setting.

Chuck pulled back the sheet to inspect her leg while I headed to retrieve the cast saw. When I returned, something had changed.

Chuck's face was blank but tense—focused, almost frozen. His eyes darted quickly from mine back to the cast, and I knew instantly that something was wrong.

I caught a whiff of it before I saw anything. The odor was unmistakable—wet, rotting, putrid. The white plaster cast had taken on a brown hue, and the stench coming from it hit us like a brick wall.

"Ma'am," Chuck asked gently, "can you tell us what happened?"

She nodded sweetly. "Oh, I broke my ankle several weeks ago—compound fracture. They had to do surgery. Then about a week ago, I was walking around my yard with my crutches, lost my footing and fell again. I couldn't get up. I laid there screaming 'til my neighbor found me and helped me back to my house. The pain increasingly got worse as the days went by.

Today, the swelling and pressure inside of my cast made it impossible for me to walk anymore so I decided to call the ambulance to take me to see the doctor."

Chuck and I exchanged a glance. This wasn't going to be a routine cast removal.

We prepped the bed with linen savers and gowned up, masking and donning eye protection like we were about to remove a live grenade. I started the saw and carefully began cutting down the centerline of the cast on the front and then we turned her on her side and cut the back of the cast. It was crusty and brittle in some places, soggy in others. Once the cuts were complete, we used the spreaders and began working the layers apart.

That's when the smell hit a whole new level.

We used bandage scissors to cut through the padding, and with every layer disturbed, the smell intensified—like a compost pile set on fire in the middle of a septic tank with a large twist of ammonia. We each grabbed a side of the cast and slowly pulled it apart.

What I saw next stopped me cold.

On the linen savers beneath her leg were tiny brown objects that began to *move*.

"Chuck," I said slowly, "is that...?"

He didn't even let me finish.

"YES IT IS."

Maggots. Not just a few. A *colony*. They were crawling up her leg, burrowing into the padding, dancing on the bed like they owned the place. And then we saw them—two small open wounds on the inside of her ankle, each one swarming with larvae, packed like sardines in a tin.

I backed away immediately and stepped through the curtain into the hallway—face pale, stomach churning—and nearly collided with our ER physician, Dr. Lupinacci.

He looked at me and raised an eyebrow. "Jimmy, what's wrong?"

I opened my mouth but my brain failed me.

"...Magnets," I muttered. "Thousands of magnets."

He blinked. "Magnets?"

I nodded solemnly. "MAGNETS."

He chuckled, patted me on the shoulder, and walked in to take a look. A second later I heard him say, "Call Dr. Moorehouse and tell him *HIS* patient is here."

I did exactly that. I called Dr. Moorehouse and explained the situation—the re-fracture, the wounds, and the maggot infestation. His response?

He let out a heavy sigh, followed by a tone that clearly suggested he wasn't exactly thrilled to be talking to me.

"As I previously instructed you, send her to X-ray. I'll be there soon."

So Chuck and I wrapped her leg in fresh linen savers, discarded the infested ones—after dousing the maggots in rubbing alcohol—and transported her off to radiology. She was still smiling, bless her heart.

When she returned, Dr. Moorehouse had arrived. He calmly opened the wrap, inspected the wounds, then turned to us and asked, "Can I have some diluted hydrogen peroxide?"

We mixed it with saline and handed it over. He poured some into the wound sites and began picking out the maggots with sterile fine-point tweezers, one by one. His hands were steady, almost routine.

After a few minutes, he examined the tissue and nodded approvingly.

"These wounds look great," he said. "Clean. No necrosis, no infection. Our little friends here did their job."

And just like that, he whisked her off to the OR to repair her fractures.

I stood there stunned. I'd been a paramedic for years and was now working full-time in the ER, but nothing—*nothing*—had prepared me for that sight. It stuck with me the rest of the day.

That evening, I left the ER to head to my night shift at the ambulance service. What I didn't know was that Chuck had already called ahead and told my crew the whole story.

Exhausted, I walked into the station and was greeted with cheerful faces and the smell of takeout.

"We got you dinner, Jimmy," one of them said, grinning. "Chinese. Extra fried rice."

I took one look, turned pale, and walked right back out shaking my head.

And to this very day, I still find myself staring at fried rice for a few minutes before taking a bite—just to make sure it doesn't suddenly start moving. True story.

29 Torch

It was a relatively quiet afternoon in the ER when a middle-aged man walked in clutching his left hand with a towel, his face contorted in pain. He had accidentally smashed his index finger with a hammer while doing some home repairs. When we unwrapped it, there was an angry, swollen hematoma pressing hard under his fingernail—purple, tight, and clearly throbbing with pressure.

Dr. Hope strolled in with his usual calm demeanor, gave it a glance, and said, "Looks like we need to relieve that pressure."

He called out his go-to supplies like a chef ordering ingredients: "Methyl ethyl chloride, saline, betadine, and a disposable cautery pen."

I gathered the items while he carefully cleaned the patient's fingertip with betadine, followed by a rinse of saline. Then, he sprayed the methyl ethyl chloride—an instant refrigerant used for numbing—over the nail. The patient winced slightly at the cold.

Without missing a beat, Dr. Hope uncapped the cautery pen, activated it, and leaned in to burn a small hole through the nail plate—standard procedure to release the pressure from a subungual hematoma.

Only, this wasn't standard.

The moment the glowing tip of the cautery pen touched the nail—WHOOSH—the man's fingernail *burst into flames.* Not just a little singe. Full-on flame. The kind that made a *whooshing* sound and danced in the air like a Fourth of July sparkler.

The patient, naturally, began waving his flaming finger around in sheer panic, yelling, "OH MY GOD! OH MY GOD!" You could hear the fire slicing through the air with each frantic motion.

Dr. Hope, eyes wide, started trying to catch the man's hand mid-air like he was wrangling a firefly with a net. "Hold still! Hold still!" he barked, ducking and lunging like he was chasing a rogue balloon.

Finally, with the precision of a practiced ER ninja, he snatched the patient's hand and plunged the blazing digit into a nearby cup of saline.

Sssssssssshhhhh.

The fire hissed out, leaving behind a smell that instantly filled the room—burning hair, scorched plastic, and maybe a touch of fried chicken skin.

We all stood there, stunned. The man's fingernail was now blackened, split straight down the middle like some cursed artifact. It looked more like a demon claw than anything human.

Dr. Hope stepped back, blinked a few times, and then deadpanned in his dry and distinct high-pitched voice:

"Well… I'm not trying' to be smart or anything, but that's not something that you get to see every day."

That did it. I had been holding back laughter through the whole flaming finger fiasco, but at that line, I couldn't take it anymore. I lost it—doubled over, gasping for breath between fits of laughter.

Even the patient, still in a daze with a smoldering digit, managed to crack a small, bewildered smile.

And somewhere in the chaos of it all, I knew this would go down as one of those ER stories we'd be telling for the rest of our careers. And maybe even write about in a book someday. And I was right!

30 Cane & Disabled

It was a typical mid-afternoon lull in the emergency department—just the kind of calm that gives ER staff that uneasy sense something ridiculous is brewing just outside the sliding glass doors.

Triage Nurse Mandy barely looked up when the next patient stepped through the automatic entrance. She could already hear the rhythmic *thump... thump... thump* of wood on tile before she saw him. A large, burly man, maybe in his late forties, was hobbling dramatically with a massive four-foot oak cane, the kind you'd expect to see in a movie, like *Walking Tall*, not an emergency department.

He groaned with each step as if death himself were latched onto his lumbar spine. The cane wasn't just a walking aid—it was his stage prop, an instrument of his performance.

"I need to see a doctor now!" he barked. "My back's killing me. I'm out of my meds—Hydrocodone. I'm hurting bad and I need them now!"

Mandy asked the standard questions—onset, history, meds, allergies. The man was vague and irritable, waving his prescription bottle like a badge of entitlement, though it was clearly empty and worn down to label shreds. His blood pressure was elevated, but not much else seemed wrong. No visible distress except the theatrics. Still, protocol dictated he be taken back for further evaluation.

He was assigned to Room 6, where Dr. Harper, one of the more seasoned ER physicians, waited with a neutral face and a clipboard that was already telling him more than the patient ever would.

"Sir," Harper said calmly, "I've reviewed your recent medical visits. Looks like you've been to five different ERs in the past three weeks for the same complaint. I'm afraid we're not going to be prescribing narcotics today."

The man blinked. The cane stopped tapping on the floor tile. For half a second, his face betrayed a flicker of "you got me," before rage took over.

"You piece of garbage!" he roared, standing—no, springing—from the stretcher with the miraculous agility of a gymnast. "You people don't care about pain! You just like watching folks suffer!"

He swung the oak cane like a war club, knocking over the small Mayo stand with a crash. A water cup went flying. A nurse peeked in and immediately turned around. As the man stormed out of the room, his limp was gone. He moved quickly and fluidly, cursing like a sailor as he shoved open the ER door with his foot.

The staff watched, stunned, as he swaggered across the lobby, forcefully pushing open the automatic sliding exit doors, and strutted to the parking lot—directly to a shiny red pickup truck parked, of course, in a handicapped space. A woman in her late sixties was walking toward the ER entrance just as the man jumped in his truck.

Without pause, he threw it into reverse.

BANG.

The truck's rear bumper struck the woman, sending her tumbling to the pavement. Gasps rang out from the lobby. Someone yelled, "Call

911!"—a bit ironic, considering they were standing in the emergency department.

The man hit the brakes, glanced back, and then hit the gas again. Tires squealed as he shot out of the lot, leaving behind a very bruised and frightened pedestrian and a lobby full of shocked witnesses.

Security got the plate number, and the police were called immediately.

Within the hour, word came back from law enforcement: they had located and arrested the man at a gas station not far from the hospital. His truck still bore traces of the collision, and in his glove compartment were dozens of empty pill bottles from multiple states—Florida, Alabama, Kentucky, Mississippi.

Turns out, the man was part of a nationwide drug-seeking ring. A small network of people who made their living—quite lucratively—by visiting emergency rooms under various names and complaints, fishing for narcotics. When successful, they paid cash to avoid pharmacy red flags, pooled their pills, and then sold them on the street.

The arresting officer said, almost in disbelief, "This guy was making more than I do. Over $150,000 a year. Just selling pills he conned out of ERs."

Back at the hospital, the woman he struck was treated for minor injuries—thankfully nothing life-threatening. Dr. Harper, meanwhile, jotted a note in the chart:

Diagnosis: Malingering with miraculous recovery upon prescription denial.

The oak cane, oddly enough, was found abandoned in the parking lot—laying there like a wooden exclamation mark punctuating the absurdity of the whole ordeal.

31 · Butt Light

It was just after 7:00 a.m. when the ER doors slid open and a lanky, balding man in his late 50s shuffled up to the triage window. He looked agitated. Restless. And he refused to sit.

Meghan Cole, a seasoned ER charge nurse, had seen it all—or so she thought.

"Good morning, sir," she said with her usual warm-but-weary tone. "What brings you in today?"

The man looked around, as if making sure no one else was within earshot, and leaned in closer.

"I stuck a candle up my ass," he said matter-of-factly.

Meghan blinked. "I'm sorry—what?"

He repeated himself slowly and slightly louder: "I said I stuck a candle up my ass."

Still trying to keep her professional face, Meghan tilted her head and asked, "Sir… why?"

He looked downright offended that she would question it. "It was my birthday yesterday. I was watching Fox News... and well, I got turned on. So I grabbed one of them glass jar candles and, you know, stuck it up there."

Meghan didn't ask what exactly on Fox News had turned him on. Some questions were better left unanswered.

She stood up from her triage chair, already reaching for gloves. "Okay, let's get you to an exam room." She looked at ER doctor Ray Jerkins on her way. It was that secret ER look that screamed – COME GO WITH ME!

She led the human candle holder back to Room 4 and had him disrobe and lie on his side. He kept trying to explain the situation—how it was one of those big three-wick candles from Walmart, the kind with inspirational words like *"Live, Laugh, Love"* printed on the label. Apparently, it didn't feel like love anymore.

Double-gloving, Meghan began to perform a careful digital rectal exam about the same time that Dr. Jerkins entered the room. Sure enough, she could feel the base of a large cylindrical object—a glass jar candle lodged firmly and deeply inside.

With a sigh, she pulled off her gloves and looked at Dr. Jerkins and told him what he probably already knew: "He has a large glass candle jar in his rectum."

X-rays and labs were done and surgery was paged. The patient was prepped, paperwork was signed, and soon enough, he was whisked upstairs to have his birthday souvenir professionally extracted.

As they wheeled him out of the ER, he looked at Meghan and said, "Maybe I should've used the smaller candle."

She just gave him a tired smile and replied, "Next year, just eat some cake."

32 A Quiet End of Always

It was just past 10 a.m. on a cloudy Tuesday when the EMS tones dropped. The dispatcher's voice crackled through the radio: *"Respond to a possible gunshot wound. Female - 40's. Self-inflicted. Husband on scene. Law enforcement enroute."*

The first unit to arrive, a seasoned paramedic crew—Dan and Marissa—entered the suburban home with their gear in tow. They moved quickly through the narrow hallway, led by a trembling police officer who had arrived moments earlier. He could only manage a whisper: *"It's bad. Real bad."*

They stepped into the bedroom and were immediately assaulted by the coppery sting of fresh blood. The walls looked like something out of a warzone—bathed in a macabre constellation of arterial spray, pink tissue, and fragments of bone. The carpet beneath their boots squished with saturation. Against the far wall, slumped in a sitting position, was the woman.

She was in her 40s. Her body still bore the shape of life, but what remained above the ears defied comprehension. Her entire cranium had been obliterated by the .357 magnum projectile. There was no skull, no visible brain, no hair, only a face. Yet somehow, impossibly, she was still breathing.

Her mouth hung slack, and with each ragged exhalation, a haunting, guttural growl escaped her lips—something primal, inhuman. Her eyes—still intact—were wide open, locked in an upward, lifeless stare. Marissa recoiled instinctively but steadied herself.

Dan, hardened by years in the field, quickly checked vitals. She had a pulse. Rapid. Thready. Blood pressure low. Respiratory effort present, but agonal. *"We need to move—now."*

They packaged her as best they could, stabilizing her airway with a nasal trumpet and applying a large abdominal dressing over the exposed cavity where her skull once was. There was no time for delicate measures. They secured her on the stretcher and rushed to the rig, the husband trailing behind them, his face soaked in tears and speckled with the blood and tissue of the woman he'd shared a life with.

At the hospital, the trauma team already alerted, the medics rolled her into Trauma Bay 2 where Dr. Page awaited. Calm, composed, and sharp as a razor, he'd seen just about everything. But even he froze for a half-second when he saw her.

He scanned the body, then the face—the empty skull—then the monitor.

"She's breathing through brainstem reflexes," he said quietly. "There's nothing left. No cerebral function. No survivability."

Still, he moved with purpose. He motioned to a nurse. "Get me the husband."

The husband, still wearing a wrinkled flannel shirt drenched in blood and brain matter, stood silently in the hallway until Dr. Page stepped out to speak with him. The man collapsed into the wall, sobbing when he heard the prognosis.

"There's nothing we can do to bring her back," Dr. Page said gently. "We can make her comfortable, and I'll make sure you have the time you need with her."

The husband's voice cracked through gasps of despair. "Please... do *something*. You have to try. You have to do everything."

Dr. Page gave a long, patient pause. He placed a steady hand on the man's shoulder. "We'll take care of her. We'll do everything we can—to give her peace."

With compassion masking finality, Dr. Page arranged for her to be cleaned and intubated. She was put on a Bird ventilator by the respiratory therapist. A nurse brought in a wide recliner chair and positioned it beside the bed. The chaplain was called. Warm blankets were laid across the woman's chest. Someone handed the husband some cleansing wipes and a gown. He took them without looking, only to kneel beside the bed, trembling hands reaching for hers.

The ventilator hissed its mechanical rhythm, each rise of her chest a cruel echo of a life that had already left. Yet the husband whispered to her for hours. Stories of their first date. Their wedding song. The last argument they had over nothing. The names of their children.

At 2:17 p.m., the monitor began its final countdown. Her oxygen saturation dropped. Blood pressure tanked. The reflexive breaths slowed, then stopped.

She passed with her husband still holding her hand, tears streaming down his cheeks, whispering *"I love you"* over and over again.

Dr. Page walked in silently, turned off the ventilator, and laid a gentle hand on the woman's shoulder. He looked to the husband and said softly, "She held on as long as she could... just for you."

The curtain was pulled closed. And the room fell quiet.

Note: This story is a dramatized account, based upon a true event. It is intended for storytelling purposes, based on scenarios that are unfortunately not uncommon in emergency medicine. It is written with the deepest respect for those affected by suicide and trauma. If you or someone you know is struggling, reach out to the Suicide & Crisis Lifeline at 988.

The Lifeline and 988

988 has been designated as the new three-digit dialing code that will route callers to the National Suicide Prevention Lifeline. While some areas may be currently able to connect to the Lifeline by dialing 988, this dialing code will be available to everyone across the United States starting on July 16, 2022.

When people call, text, or chat 988, they will be connected to trained counselors that are part of the existing National Suicide Prevention Lifeline network. These trained counselors will listen, understand how their problems are affecting them, provide support, and connect them to resources if necessary.

The current Lifeline phone number (1-800-273-8255) will always remain available to people in emotional distress or suicidal crisis, even after 988 is launched nationally.

The Lifeline's network of over 200 crisis centers has been in operation since 2005, and has been proven to be effective. It's the counselors at these local crisis centers who answer the contacts the Lifeline receives every day. Numerous studies have shown that callers feel less suicidal, less depressed, less overwhelmed and more hopeful after speaking with a Lifeline counselor.

33 CODE COPENHAGEN

Zack Marden was a seasoned ER nurse who had worked nearly every corner of the emergency department over the years. Smart, calm under pressure, and always quick with a sarcastic comment, Zack had earned his reputation as a natural leader. When he accepted the role of night shift Associate Director, no one was surprised—he was the kind of guy who could coordinate a trauma, de-escalate a combative psych patient, and troubleshoot a broken bedside monitor all in one shift… with a can of Copenhagen in his back pocket.

But like all great ER legends, Zack's most famous story wasn't about the time he saved someone's life. No, it was about the time *his* life was (allegedly) lost—right there in his own office.

It was a slow stretch at Westside Hospital. Ambulance traffic had been light, walk-ins even lighter. The ER staff hadn't needed Zack's help in weeks, so he busied himself in his office catching up on scheduling, quality performance paperwork, and the latest stack of admin nonsense someone thought was important.

That night, around 2 a.m., Zack sat at his desk with the glow of his monitor casting a soft light across the room. A lip full of wintergreen Copenhagen was tucked neatly in place, and a half-empty bottle of Diet Dr. Pepper sat beside his keyboard. As the lull of night settled in, so did Zack. Slouched in his office chair, arms folded across his chest, the soft whispering sound of the HVAC became a lullaby.

And then he was out. Just like that.

What no one knew—Zack included—was that he had recently developed narcolepsy. He hadn't made the connection yet. He just thought he was "burned out" or "running on fumes." But that night, his body gave in. As he fell into an unplanned nap, his head tilted slightly to the side. The wad of dip in his mouth began to slowly leach down the corner of his lips, pooling into a small, grotesque puddle of brown sludge on his shirt.

It wasn't until around 3:15 a.m. when Sarah, one of the ER techs, wandered in to ask Zack about the staff schedule. The door was cracked. She knocked. No answer. She peeked in—and froze.

There was Zack, completely still. Slumped. Pale. Brown liquid seeping from his mouth. Eyes barely open. It looked like a combination of a stroke, GI bleed, and death itself.

She screamed.

"ZACK IS DEAD!"

Her voice echoed down the ER entry hall. In seconds, the charge nurse dropped her chart, and the crew stormed into Zack's office like Navy SEALs on a hostage rescue. A portable monitor and crash cart were being pushed in when Steve, one of the night nurses, shouted, "Zack, buddy?! ZACK?!"

No response.

So he did what any ER nurse with poor impulse control might do in a moment of adrenaline-fueled panic—he punched Zack square in the chest.

Zack's eyes flew open as he let out a startled, raspy *"What the hell!?"*

He looked around, bewildered by the crowd in his office and the heart monitor leads being waved near his face. He wiped his mouth with the back of his hand, only to smear dip juice across his cheek.

"Am I… dying?" he asked.

Steve, laughing, backed up. "Dying? You looked like you'd been dead for two hours, man! What the hell is that stuff coming out of your face?"

Zack blinked. "Copenhagen."

For weeks afterward, staff would knock on Zack's office door with mock concern.

"You still with us, big guy?"

"Need a pulse check, or you good?"

A new "emergency alert" sign was put on the whiteboard simply said: Check Zack—q 1 hour.

Eventually, after a few more episodes of daytime "nodding off," Zack followed up with a sleep specialist and was diagnosed with narcolepsy. He adjusted his lifestyle, took his meds, and the episodes faded into memory. But the story lived on.

To this day, new hires are told: “Don’t go to Zack’s office alone. If he’s got dip in and isn’t moving—assess first, punch later.”

And Zack? He just smiles and shakes his head whenever someone stops by and asks, “You still alive, boss?”

Because in the ER, your worst moment sometimes become your most legendary.

34 Pain in the Neck

The call came in just after 10:30 p.m. on a cool Friday night. A teenage girl was enroute via EMS after a motor vehicle accident on one of those notorious South Alabama back roads where sharp curves and reckless youth made a dangerous cocktail. From the limited radio report, we knew she was critical, recalled ER Nurse, Steve Hartman. The medics mentioned something about a "foreign body to the neck" and "severe facial trauma." That was enough to call in the trauma team and page Dr. Conner Charleston, the on-call general surgeon, before the ambulance even pulled in.

The girl arrived on a backboard, blood pooling along her right side and a bizarre, glinting chrome object protruding from the left side of her neck. The real showstopper, though, was her right eye—protruding from its socket like a surrealist painting come to life. She was awake but quiet, her breathing labored and wet, her good eye darting around, frantic and aware.

Nobody said a word for a moment—nurses, techs, even the seasoned paramedics stood there momentarily frozen. It wasn't the blood. They'd all seen worse. It was the sheer absurdity of the mechanism of injury—the angle, the eyeball, the foreign object that no one could quite identify yet.

We quickly got to work. IVs in both arms. Oxygen on. C-collar in place. The monitor blipped to life. Her blood pressure was low but holding. She was young, and young people compensate like warriors. But the clock was ticking.

X-ray techs were called stat. In the days before CT scans, they did what they could with plain films and clinical hunches. When the images were developed and clipped up to the backlit board, everyone leaned in.

And that's when Dr. Charleston walked in.

He was a calm and gentle man, but he was never one to sugarcoat a thing. He glanced at the film, then leaned back slightly with a look of genuine disbelief. He jabbed a finger at the film and let out a short bark of a laugh.

"Ain't THAT some shit," he said.

And he wasn't wrong.

The X-ray told the whole story in one horrifying still frame. A metal rod—the gear shift lever from an old manual transmission truck—had entered the girl's neck on the left, just above the clavicle. It traversed the soft tissues of her neck, slipped across her trachea, and angled up under the orbital floor on the right. The pressure from the metal bar had literally pushed the right eyeball out of its socket. Miraculously, it had stopped just shy of exiting through the right temple. If you looked closely at her right hairline, you could see the faintest bulge.

But it got worse. Dr. Charleston picked up a laryngoscope and carefully inserted it down her throat. He paused and motioned for Steve to take a look.

There, gleaming in the beam of the scope like chrome jewelry at the back of her airway, was the handle of the shift lever—cutting across her trachea like some kind of mechanical bridge.

How was she still breathing?

How was she still *alive*?

The story, when it was finally pieced together, was tragic and unbelievable. She'd been on a date with a local boy, riding shotgun in his pickup. He took a curve too fast, lost control, and slammed the truck into a light pole. It was one of those old vehicles with the three-on-the-tree gearshift, mounted to the steering column. When they hit the pole, her body was thrown across the cab with brutal force. She didn't hit the dash. She hit the shifter. It impaled her like a medieval lance.

The boy had only minor injuries—broken wrist, some bruises. He'd tried to hold her upright until EMS arrived, terrified and sobbing.

Back in the ER, there were decisions to be made. Fast ones. Dr. Charleston knew this wasn't something to be delicately explored. It had to be handled in the OR—controlled setting, airway secured, vascular access ready, and everyone prepared for catastrophic hemorrhage the moment that shifter came out.

They rushed her to surgery.

The ER staff patiently waited.

And waited.

And then finally—Dr. Charleston emerged from the OR around 3 a.m. and he came by the ER, pulling off his surgical cap and running a tired hand through his thinning hair as he sat down in a chair at the nurse's station.

"She's stable," he said. "She lost the right eye, and her airway's going to be a mess for a while, but she's going to live."

There were sighs of relief and a few quiet fist bumps.

That girl became a kind of legend in our ER. Not because she survived, but because of how close she came to not surviving.

To this day, if you ask any of the old guard about the craziest X-ray they've ever seen, someone will mention the girl with the gear shifter.

35 Runaway Chariot

It was a typical day in the ER—controlled chaos, ringing alarms, and the occasional security call for an unruly patient on the adult psychiatric floor. Amid the madness, nurses Mixie Becker and Mandy Lee were tasked with discharging Mr. Earle Randall, a bilateral amputee regular who had come in earlier for minor respiratory complaints. He was stable, cleared for discharge, and eager to get home.

"Alright, Mr. Randall," Mixie said, giving his wheelchair a slight push as they navigated the hallways. "Your ride should be here any minute."

"Hope so," he muttered. "I got better things to do than sit in this place."

Mandy chuckled. "We hear that a lot."

The two nurses wheeled him through the sliding glass doors and under the ambulance bay, which overlooked the steepest driveway in the entire city. The hospital engineers had designed it that way for reasons no one quite understood, but it made for a precarious waiting spot for discharged patients.

"Let's park you right here," Mixie said, as they positioned him at the top of the hill.

As Mixie proceeded to stop the momentum of the wheelchair, however, without warning, both of the rubber hand grips on the wheelchair handles slipped right off in her hands. The sudden loss of control sent Mr. Randall rolling forward.

"Uh—Mandy?"

"What?"

The wheelchair lurched. The brakes weren't locked.

"Oh, shit—"

Gravity took over.

Mr. Randall's wheelchair shot down the steep hill like a rocket, picking up speed with every second. His arms flailed as he let out a string of curses, rolling across the driveway, and directly into the road.

"STOP THE CHAIR!" Mixie shouted as she and Mandy took off in a dead sprint.

The chair hit the curb, launching him into the air like a scene straight out of an action movie.

With an unceremonious thud, he landed face-up on the well-manicured lawn of the neighboring property.

Mixie and Mandy finally caught up, panting, staring down at the man they had just—accidentally—launched from hospital care straight into someone's front yard.

"You okay, Mr. Randall?" Mandy wheezed, leaning over.

Earle blinked up at them, took a deep breath, and exhaled.

"Well, that was a hell of a ride," he said. "I am fine! Can we pretend that never happened?"

Mixie and Mandy exchanged a glance.

"Deal," Mixie said, helping him up.

Just then, his ride pulled up—a rusted old van with a bumper barely hanging on. The driver gave them a suspicious look but said nothing as they loaded Mr. Randall inside.

As the van drove off, Mandy turned to Mixie.

"I too say we *never* speak of this again."

Mixie nodded. "Agreed."

And with that, they walked—briskly—back into the ER, pretending nothing had ever happened.

36 DON'T RELAX THAT MUCH

Chuck Crawford and Zack Marden were seasoned ER nurses—gritty, efficient, and cool under pressure. They worked in a busy emergency department that regularly received transfers from rural hospitals, often sending them what they couldn't manage. On this particular afternoon, the report was brief but serious: a STEMI coming from a tiny, under-equipped critical access hospital about 45 minutes out. The patient was a 68-year-old Vietnam veteran, with chest pain, classic ECG changes, and a nitro drip enroute. ETA: 10 minutes.

Chuck stood at the nurse's station reviewing his setup checklist. Zack was beside him, adjusting the cardiac monitor and prepping necessary supplies.

The ambulance finally rolled into the bay and paramedics wheeled in a lanky, weathered man with a long gray beard, faded fatigues, and a look of deep unease. His name was Russell Kinley, and his eyes darted nervously around the room, scanning monitors, wires, and hands.

“You must be the A-team,” he said, trying to smile but not quite pulling it off.

Chuck leaned in with his usual laid-back demeanor. “Hey man, don’t you worry—you’re in great hands. Zack and I are going to take good care of you. And let me give you a piece of advice, you cannot get excited until I get excited.”

Russell exhaled like he’d been holding his breath for the last hour. “Okay,” he said, nodding. “Well, that makes me feel better. Thank you. I think I’ll just lay back and relax while you guys do your job.”

Zack gave him a reassuring pat on the arm. “Sounds like a plan.”

They got to work—placing leads, checking vitals, assessing the IV drips, updating labs, pulling up the Cath lab protocol, and beginning what felt like the longest transfer packet paperwork in the history of medicine. Chuck flipped through half-legible copies of rural documentation while Zack typed in orders and input medical history from the sheet handed over by the medics.

Then, without warning, a sharp and rapid *BEEP* broke through the controlled hum of the ER.

Both men turned in unison toward the monitor.

"V-Tach," Zack said immediately, his voice cutting through the noise.

Russell was lying back with his eyes closed—completely unresponsive.

"Russell!" Chuck barked, grabbing the man's shoulder and shaking him firmly. "Russell, wake up!" No response.

Zack was already reaching for the defibrillator. "Shock him, Chuck!"

Chuck didn't hesitate. He grabbed the paddles, charged the unit, called out, "Clear!" and pushed the buttons.

The jolt lit up the man's chest and cracked the tension in the room like a lightning strike.

Almost instantly, Russell's eyes popped open. He stared straight at them and croaked, "Don't do that again!"

Chuck blinked, half shocked himself, then glanced at the monitor.

Sinus rhythm. Perfect.

Zack gave a relieved laugh, trying to mask the adrenaline still rushing through him. “Well, damn. That was effective.”

Chuck smiled and leaned down toward the veteran, who was now blinking at the ceiling, mildly irritated but very much alive. “It’s okay for you to relax, Russell,” Chuck said with a grin, “but don’t relax *that* much again.”

The man chuckled, then winced at the pain in his chest. “Roger that, Chief.”

Minutes later, the Cath lab team arrived and wheeled Russell away for intervention. Chuck and Zack stood side by side, silent for a moment, watching the stretcher disappear down the hallway.

“Think he’ll be okay?” Zack asked.

Chuck exhaled slowly. "He survived the jungle. He survived this. I think he'll be fine."

Zack nodded and reached for the next stack of transfer paperwork. "Still," he said, "I vote we put a *Do Not Chill Too Hard* wristband on the next guy."

Chuck laughed. "Add that to the protocol. Right under *Notify Cath lab* and *try not to die in triage.*"

Another shift, another life saved, another tale for the ER lore—one where a Vietnam vet flirted with death for a moment, just long enough to be shocked back to life by a pair of ER nurses with steady hands and a sharp sense of humor.

37 JOHN 15:13

It was a late afternoon when the call came over the radio: cardiac arrest inbound from a rural EMS agency, estimated arrival time five minutes. The tone of the county dispatcher's voice carried an edge—urgent, strained, as if even she could feel something was off.

Inside the ER, the announcement sparked an instant wave of preparation. Nurses snapped on gloves, the respiratory therapist prepped airway supplies, and the physician on duty—a seasoned ER doc named Dr. Hensley—called for the crash cart to be staged and ready. The ER team flowed onto the ambulance dock like a well-oiled machine, positioning themselves at the ready.

The ambulance appeared around the corner of the bay, backing up faster than usual, tires squealing slightly as the driver struggled to guide it into place. Something about the way it approached didn't feel right. The back of the rig tilted slightly as it stopped hard against the bumpers. The ER staff instinctively braced themselves.

One of the nurses, Dana, stepped forward and pulled open the back doors of the ambulance.

What she saw made her gasp.

There, strapped to the stretcher, was a lifeless patient—ashen, unmoving, and clearly pulseless. But it wasn't just the patient.

Slumped on the floor beside the stretcher was another body. A paramedic. Motionless. Face pale, lips blue.

For a moment, time froze.

"Get help out here!" Dana screamed, turning back toward the ER entrance.

People flooded forward. More nurses, techs, another physician. It took just seconds for the scene to explode into motion.

Two stretchers were wheeled in—one for the original patient, one for the medic. CPR began immediately on both as they were separated and rushed inside.

The driver, a wide-eyed EMT named Keith, stood on the dock in stunned silence. His voice cracked as he explained, "I didn't know—he was doing compressions... he told me to drive fast... I never heard him stop... I thought... I thought he was still working him..."

His voice trailed off as the weight of it all settled over the team.

Inside Trauma Room 1, the ER team worked frantically on the original patient, but he was gone—too far gone. No pulse, no signs of life, no chance. In Trauma Room 2, they worked just as hard on the medic—trying to bring back one of their own.

His name was Brent, 52 years old. A father. A volunteer paramedic. He had left his day job at the feed store that afternoon when the tones dropped, because that's what he always did. Rural EMS didn't have a deep bench. If Brent didn't show up, no one would.

Dr. Hensley stood at the foot of Brent's bed as the monitor flatlined and the final decision had to be made.

"Time of death, 17:42," he said quietly.

The room fell into silence. No one spoke. No one moved.

The tragedy hit harder than most. Not just because two lives were lost, but because of *how* it happened. Brent had died doing chest compressions on someone he never even knew. Alone in the back of a speeding ambulance, working tirelessly with no one to notice when he collapsed. No backup. No relief.

Just him, the patient, and his last act of service.

Later, as the story spread through the hospital and across county lines, the silence gave way to somber reflection. The question was raised repeatedly—*How could this happen?*

But in rural EMS, this was the reality. Departments staffed with volunteers. One EMT to drive. One paramedic in back. Old equipment, sometimes - long transport times, and the unrelenting weight of doing more with less.

They weren't doing it for the money—there wasn't any.

They weren't doing it for recognition—there was none.

They did it because someone had to.

Brent became a symbol of something many had long taken for granted: the invisible backbone of rural emergency medicine. A man who gave everything—*literally everything*—to serve his community.

A candlelight vigil was held in the town square that weekend. People came from every neighboring county. Fire trucks lined the streets. Flags were lowered. And in the center of it all, someone placed Brent's helmet on top of a stretcher, draped in black, with a note pinned to it that read: ***"Greater love has no one than this, than to lay down one's life for his friends."*** — *John 15:13 (NKJV)*

Rural EMS may operate in the shadows of big-city systems, but its light burns no less bright.

And sometimes, it burns so fiercely that it gives all it has—until there's nothing left.

38 Splash Down

It was a perfectly calm morning in the emergency department at Medical Center East—for now.

The sound of the monitors, the ding of a telemetry alarm, and the occasional cough from a curtained room were the only sounds filling the ER at 9 a.m. The lull wouldn't last. It never did.

Meghan Cole, the ER charge nurse, and only female staff member for that particular day shift, was sipping bad coffee and reviewing her patient board when she heard the unmistakable sound of boots on tile.

Two uniformed city police officers walked through the ambulance bay doors escorting a woman in handcuffs. She was dressed in pajama pants, flip-flops, and a stretched-out tank top that hadn't seen a washing machine in months. Her hair was matted, her eyes jittery, and her mouth never stopped moving.

"She started complaining of chest pain in the back seat," one of the officers said. "Per policy, we've got to get her cleared before we can book her."

Meghan nodded. She'd seen it all—drunks, brawlers, meth heads with hearts that beat like hummingbirds. Nothing fazed her anymore.

The patient was placed on a stretcher in Room 4, still cuffed. Meghan went in to start triage and vitals. "Ma'am, I need to ask you a few questions about your pain."

The woman clutched her chest dramatically and rocked back and forth. "It's bad. Real bad. Like, right in the middle here—hurts so bad I can't hardly breathe."

"On a scale of one to ten?" Meghan asked dryly.

"Fifteen!" the woman replied, eyes wide. "I think I'm dying."

Before Meghan could finish entering the triage note, the woman twisted slightly and said, "Um, hey... I need to use the bathroom, like I need to go right this minute."

Meghan peered at her and said, "Okay, but since you're under arrest, we can't leave you alone in the restroom. I'll have to go in with you."

The woman nodded eagerly. "That's fine. I just gotta go really bad."

Meghan escorted her down the hall to the single restroom and followed her in, propping the door open with a trash can just enough so the officers standing outside could see the movement inside.

"I'm in here with you, but I'm not watching," Meghan said flatly. "Just do your thing."

The woman sat down on the toilet, sighed—and then it happened.

CLINK. TINK-TINK-TINK-SPLASH.

The unmistakable sound of glass hitting porcelain.

Meghan turned around. She blinked once. Then again. Floating awkwardly in the toilet bowl was a small, very real, very used crack pipe.

The woman's eyes locked with Meghan's. Her pupils were the size of pencil tips. Her mouth hung open. But somehow, she still had the audacity to say:

"That's not mine."

And on cue, Meghan didn't miss a beat.

"Well honey," she said coolly, "since there are only two of us in here, and I'm pretty damn sure it's not *mine*, I'd say it must be *yours*."

The patient's eyes darted to the pipe. She looked like a raccoon caught raiding a trash can. Meghan gently helped her off the toilet, turned off the light, and opened the door.

The two officers were standing just outside, arms crossed. Before Meghan could say a word, the patient blurted out in full-volume:

"THAT NURSE DROPPED HER CRACK PIPE IN THE TOILET!"

Meghan froze. One of the officers blinked. The other smirked.

"Ma'am," said the smirking one, "I've known Meghan Cole for 12 years. If she's smoking' crack, then I'm really a high school cheerleader named Tiffany."

The other officer leaned in, looked into the toilet, then at Meghan. "You want to file that as evidence or should we just count it as an extra drug charge?"

Meghan, still composed, replied, "Bag it. It's medical waste now—but it's also Exhibit A."

The patient was taken back to Room 4 for a full cardiac workup—normal EKG, normal vitals, no distress unless someone said the word *jail.* After her release, she was finally cleared for transport to the city holding facility… minus one vaginally concealed crack pipe.

Later that afternoon, while in the break room, Meghan recounted the moment with a shake of her head and a half-smile.

"You know," she said to one of her co-workers, "I became a nurse to make a difference. Now I can identify a crack pipe by the high-pitch sound it makes when it bounces off a toilet bowl after being released from a vagina. What a time to be alive."

39 WHERE IS IT COMING FROM?

It was just after sunrise in the ER. The overnight storm had cleared, leaving a gray haze hanging over the hospital. Inside, the day shift was just starting to settle in with coffee, light jokes, and the anticipation of whatever craziness might walk—or roll—through the doors that morning.

The calm was interrupted by a radio call from rural EMS.

"Medic 7 is enroute to your facility with an adult female patient. Severe bleeding, ETA 10 minutes."

Steve Hartman, an ER nurse-paramedic with years under his belt and a sixth sense for chaos, picked up the receiver. "Copy that," he replied, pressing the transmit button. "Where's she bleeding from?"

There was a pause on the other end.

"Say again?"

Steve repeated himself, slower this time. "Where... is... the bleeding... coming from?"

The EMS crew answered confidently.

"Geneva."

Steve stared at the radio for a moment, his lips parted in disbelief. "Roger that," he said dryly, rubbing his forehead. "We'll see you when you get here."

He hung up the receiver and shook his head. "Apparently the bleeding is coming from *Geneva.* Not her nose, not her leg. Just Geneva."

Ten minutes later, the ambulance backed into the dock and the patient was wheeled inside. She was an older woman in her sixties, frail and pale, with a blanket wrapped around her lower half. She winced as the stretcher bumped through the ER doors. The medic gave a quick, vague report, reiterating only that she was "bleeding bad" and "hurting down there."

Marilyn McKissack, ER Director and longtime nurse, led the way to Room 3. She was no stranger to bizarre injuries, awkward moments, or anatomy-defying stories, but something about this case felt different.

Inside the room, Marilyn pulled the curtain shut and began assessing the patient. She gently helped the woman out of her clothes and into a gown.

And then everything changed.

"Steve!" she called from the room, her voice laced with disbelief. "You need to come see this. You are *not* going to believe it."

Steve walked in, still sipping his coffee, but that sip stopped midway as soon as he saw what Marilyn had uncovered.

Protruding from the woman's vaginal opening was a long, coiled section of bowel. It looked dusky, dry in some places, and faintly hemorrhaging from irritated tissue. The patient laid calmly, breathing slowly, eyes half-closed like she'd just been mildly inconvenienced by a nosebleed.

Steve blinked. "Is that…?"

"Bowel," Marilyn confirmed. "Coming from... yeah. That's where the bleeding is coming from."

Steve carefully knelt beside the patient. "Ma'am, how long has this been going on?"

She shrugged. "Couple days, I reckon."

He paused. "And why didn't you come to the hospital sooner?"

"I don't have a ride," she replied flatly.

Steve stared at her for a second. "But... you called EMS today."

"Well," she said, "I didn't think it was an emergency until now."

He stood slowly, speechless.

Marilyn broke the silence. "Well, it's an emergency *now,* alright."

The next hour became a flurry of activity. The on-call surgeon was paged, labs were rushed, and arrangements were made to get her to the OR. But even in the chaos, the surreal nature of the case lingered.

By the time the patient was stabilized and enroute to surgery, the story had already begun to ripple through the ER. The phrase *"Where's it coming from?"* became the quote of the day, closely followed by *"Geneva!"*

Cindy Griffin made a makeshift sign for the nurse's station:
"Hey Steve, Where is the bleeding coming from?"

And though the day moved on and other patients came and went, the image of that morning never quite left the minds of those who were there.

It was a classic tale of a rural community—where transportation is scarce, emergencies are optional, and you truly *never* know what they will bring you next.

But one thing was certain: Steve Hartman would never ask "Where's the bleeding coming from?" the same way again.

40 Beam us up Scotty

Another sleepy night in the ED.

The fluorescent lights buzzed low overhead, and the air carried a strange mix of floor wax and vanilla coffee. We were between patients—Amanda Powers, RN was scrolling on her phone, and Zack Marden, RN was halfway through a vending machine burrito that he would probably regret in about ten minutes. The calm before the storm, they called it.

Right on cue, the radio crackled to life. Dispatch monotoned, *"EMS inbound with a male, approx. 40s, found walking through the McDonald's drive-thru on foot attempting to order some food. Alert but altered."*

Zack and Amanda exchanged glances.

"Alert but altered," Amanda repeated, raising an eyebrow. "This is so, Tuesday."

Zack inhaled the rest of his burrito and pulled on gloves as they awaited their new patient. Moments later, the bay doors whooshed open, and in rolled

EMS—followed by not one, but two fire crews and at least four PD officers, all of them grinning like they'd just left a comedy club.

That's never a good sign.

The guy on the stretcher looked uninjured but wild-eyed. He had on a tattered T-shirt with something vaguely sci-fi on it, mismatched shoes, and a forehead sweatband he wore like a crown. As the stretcher clicked to a stop in the trauma bay 3, he sat up with sudden purpose.

"You can't keep me here," he boomed, dramatically scanning the room. "I am *Commander Vek'tal of the Klingon Empire*. And if you try to imprison me, I will FIGHT for my HONOR!"

Zack froze for a beat.

Amanda looked at him like she had just opened a dishwasher full of snakes. "WTF?"

But Zack... understood. Deeply.

He stepped closer and whispered, "Amanda, he thinks he's in *Star Trek*. And since we're all wearing blue scrubs, he thinks we're Andoorians."

She blinked. "What the hell is an Andoorian?"

"They're the blue ones with antennae. He thinks we're enemies."

She rolled her eyes so hard Zack thought they'd fall out of her head. "Great."

Still, protocol is protocol. We gently guided him back onto the stretcher, reassured him we were not, in fact, there to dishonor his house, and started our work. Zack called over one of the fire medics to help keep him still while he went for the IV, and Amanda moved to the other side to get the EKG leads in place.

He kept muttering things like *"The Federation is a lie!"* and *"I know a Romulan spy when I see one!"*

"Steady," Zack said under his breath, sliding the tourniquet in place.

Then it happened.

Like a phaser blast on stun, he lunged—not at Zack—but toward Amanda. Fast. Sudden. Intentional.

Now, Zack said "I'd love to tell you I assessed the situation, considered my options, and took swift, calculated action. But what I *did* was grab the first thing I could reach."

His trapezius muscle. The Vulcan Nerve Pinch!

I locked my hand around it and squeezed like he was a replicant gone rogue. Amanda yelped and stumbled backward, avoiding what we later realized was an attempted lip lock—apparently Commander Vek'tal had fallen hard for Nurse Amanda of the Ice Moon.

PD and fire crew moved in fast. One medic held the patient's legs, another helped untangle Amanda's EKG wires, and someone turned off the monitor alarm that had started screaming.

I was still holding him in the Vulcan Death Pinch.

"Zack," Amanda said gently, trying not to spook him. "Zack… you can let go now. I'm okay. He's turning blue."

Zack looked down. Sure enough, he was.

"Well," Zack said, slowly easing his grip, "I figured he'd like to be Andoorian like the rest of us."

Everyone in the room burst into laughter, even a couple of the cops. Amanda shot him a *seriously?* look, but he could tell she was trying not to smile.

Commander Vek'tal who was conscious and unharmed, laid back and mumbled, "Puj'..." indicating that Zack was weak.

That night, Amanda Googled "Andoorian." She still doesn't forgive me for the mental image.

They gave him fluids, ran labs, checked tox screens, and eventually sedated him just enough to keep him from starting an intergalactic war with the night shift. Turned out he'd taken something synthetic—bath salts, spice, who knows—and his mind went warp speed straight into the final frontier.

By morning, the crew had dubbed them as the *USS Andorian.* Amanda was promoted to Science Officer. Zack was the Security Chief.

And the next time someone came in speaking Klingon, Zack promised Amanda that he would not initiate a Vulcan death grip ever again.

Unless, of course, they try to kiss Amanda. Then all bets were off.

41 THE COVENANT

It was one of those deceptively calm Saturdays in the ER—clear skies, no holidays, no major events in town. The quiet buzz of fluorescent lights and the occasional beeping of monitors filled the small local hospital emergency department where Marilyn McKissack and Susan Jernigan Deal worked side by side. With only the two of them on duty and Dr. Jimmy Jones covering as the ER physician, they knew they'd have to handle anything that came through the door with grit and teamwork.

Marilyn McKissack – ER Nurse
Marilyn McKissack was the kind of nurse every patient wished they had and every hospital prayed to keep. A pillar of strength in the emergency department, she combined clinical skill with unmatched compassion. Years of experience had sharpened her instincts, yet her heart remained tender and fiercely devoted to those she served. Whether it was a child with a broken arm or a trauma patient clinging to life, Marilyn had a way of making people feel seen, safe, and cared for—even in their worst moments. Calm under pressure, quick-thinking, and deeply

intuitive, Marilyn was also the nurse others turned to when chaos reigned. Resourceful and relentless, she didn't just care for patients—she advocated for them, fought for them, and stood by them, no matter the odds.

Susan Jernigan Deal – ER Nurse

Susan Deal was a bright light in a place often shrouded in shadows. As an ER nurse, she was known for her unwavering focus, sharp clinical skills, and her warm, reassuring presence. She was the kind of nurse who remembered not only what medications a patient needed, but how they took their coffee or which side they preferred to lie on. Colleagues admired her calm demeanor, her efficiency, and her ability to find moments of grace in even the most tragic situations. She had the heart of a caregiver and the strength of a warrior—never flinching in the face of trauma, always ready to jump in, lead, and lift others up. Behind every measured action was a woman who deeply loved her work, her patients, and the people she worked beside.

Dr. Jimmy Jones – ER Physician

Dr. Jimmy Jones was the anchor of the emergency room—steady, unshakable, and wise beyond measure. Known for his hands-on approach and cool-headed leadership, he carried the burden of critical decision-making with quiet confidence. He didn't speak often unless it mattered, and when he did, people listened. A true clinician at heart, Dr. Jones blended textbook knowledge with real-world grit. He had seen the worst that humanity and nature could bring, and still chose to serve with grace and humility. Patients respected him. Nurses trusted him. And when lives were on the line, there was no one better to have at the head of the stretcher. Beneath his calm exterior was a deep well of compassion—one that guided every diagnosis, every stitch, and every difficult conversation with a grieving family.

Together, Marilyn, Susan, and Dr. Jones were more than just coworkers. They were a formidable team—battle-tested, heart-driven, and forever ready for whatever came through the doors.

Shortly after noon, the radio crackled to life with the unmistakable voice of a rural EMS crew. Marilyn picked up the receiver, her expression sharpening as she listened.

"Medic 1 is enroute with a pediatric trauma, MVC, approximately 30 miles out. One child. Critical. Multiple trauma. Mother and three siblings DOA at the scene."

The room went silent for a breath.

Marilyn and Susan locked eyes. No words were needed. Both had heard the same tone in that medic's voice—the controlled urgency of someone doing everything they could to save a child who might not make it.

As the rural EMS unit roared towards the hospital—about 30 miles away—the grim details unfurled. The accident involved a mother and her four children, bound for the local airport where they hoped to reunite with the father, who was returning from an extended overseas military deployment. EMS reported catastrophic trauma: shattered bodies, severe amputations, and injuries that defied hope.

In that suspended moment, when time seemed to bend inwards, Marilyn immediately set into motion the chain of emergency protocols. With a calm urgency, she called for backup from the hospital supervisor, her voice firm despite the pounding of her own heart.

Within minutes, the emergency department transformed. Beds were rearranged, supplies rushed from storerooms, and every available hand was thrown into the overwhelming work ahead. Outside, sirens screamed in the distance; inside, a palpable dread mixed with determined resolve.

Susan moved swiftly, prepping Trauma Room 1 with practiced precision—trauma packs, airway setup, crash cart unlocked, fluids spiked and hanging. Dr. Jones scrubbed in, reviewing pediatric protocols while also making calls to alert the on-call surgical team. They all moved like a unit—disciplined and fluid, though an unspoken dread that pulsed beneath the surface.

Minutes later, the ambulance backed up to the bay, doors flying open to reveal the mangled, bloodied form of a young boy no older than eight. His shirt was soaked in blood, one leg twisted unnaturally, facial trauma visible even under the oxygen mask. A small stuffed bear, blood-soaked and clinging to a shred of his shirt, told the story no child should ever be part of.

"Mom and three siblings... all gone," the paramedic choked out. "Dad's flying into the local airport from an extended overseas deployment. They were meeting him at the airport."

Susan's hand paused for just a second on the child's arm, her eyes welling but her body refusing to stop. The ER transformed into organized chaos. The smell of antiseptics mixed with the metallic scent of blood. Gauze soaked red. Vitals monitored. Fluids pushed. X-rays taken. Intubation performed. Fractures stabilized.

The room looked like a war zone, the kind Dr. Jones had seen in his residency rotations and unfortunately many times afterward—blood pooling, discarded trauma shears on the floor, surgical wrappers fluttering like flags of surrender. But there was no surrender. Not that day.

Against all odds, they stabilized the boy. His pulse returned to near-normal. His blood pressure responded to volume. His airway was secure. They had a fighting chance.

Then came the next blow.

Marilyn was at the nurse's station when the registration clerk walked over, pale and trembling.

"There's a man in the waiting room," she whispered. "Says he just got in from Germany. Military. He thinks his family is here."

Marilyn's heart sank. She walked slowly to Dr. Jones, then to Susan, who had just stepped back to strip off a pair of blood-soaked gloves.

The father, desperate and bereaved, had been brought into the ER by a police officer from the airport. His eyes, red and hollow, spoke of an anguish that no words could capture. Together, Marilyn, Susan, and Dr. Jones approached him—a moment suspended between duty and human compassion—as they prepared to deliver the unspeakable news.

Dr. Jones spoke first. His voice was steady, but the words landed like bricks.

"There's no easy way to say this, sir… but your wife and three of your children didn't survive the accident. We have one of your sons here with us and we have managed to stabilize his injuries.....he's alive. He's in critical condition, but stable at the moment. We're prepping him for surgery now."

The man collapsed into the chair behind him, sobbing so deeply that even Susan had to look away. When he finally stood, he asked only one thing.

"Can I see him?"

Under those harsh fluorescent lights of the ER, the father was led to the ER bed that so gently cradled the broken body of his son. His sorrow was a heavy, tangible presence that filled the room, as he painstakingly identified the remnants of a life once whole.

The man leaned down, took his son's small hand in his own, and whispered words only the two of them would ever hear.

Outside the door, Marilyn and Susan stood in silence. Susan, her voice barely audible, turned to Marilyn and said, "If anything like this ever happens to me, please... don't let my family see me like that." It was a fragile echo of vulnerability that belied her resilient exterior.

Marilyn didn't respond. She didn't need to. She only nodded.

One week later, on a rather quiet Saturday night, tragedy struck again. The local EMS was dispatched to a one-vehicle rollover on a winding backroad. The car was found mangled, halfway down an embankment.

The city communications center dispatcher's voice rang out with eerie familiarity: "Rescue 1, Engine 1 – respond to a single-vehicle rollover, three occupants. Bystanders report major trauma and one possible fatality.

Steve Hartman, ER nurse-paramedic, was on duty with Dr. Cochran. The ER was quiet when the paramedic on scene, Rocky Robbins, called in to report the status of the patients.

"We've got one coming to you with moderate multiple trauma, another one going across town to East, and… one DOA left on scene—Steve, she's one of yours."

Steve furrowed his brow. "What do you mean, one of ours?"

The Rocky's voice was hesitant.

"It's Susan Deal."

Steve dropped the phone.

The room spun.

With trembling hands, he picked it up again and immediately dialed Marilyn at home.

She answered on the second ring.

"Marilyn," Steve said, his voice breaking, "It's Susan. She was a backseat passenger in a bad MVC tonight. She didn't make it."

There was only silence on the line… followed by a whispered, "No."

Years later, Marilyn recalls remembering every detail of that fateful phone call. She remembered sitting on the sofa at her home, replaying Susan's words in her head. And now, with unbearable irony, it had happened.

Susan never got the chance to grow old. She never had the opportunity to sit in a quiet moment and tell the story of the little boy who survived because she fought so hard to keep him alive. But Marilyn did. And every time she tells the story, she remembers the weight of Susan's whisper.

And to this very day, she honors it and she will never forget it.

For those who knew Susan—those who stood beside her in the chaos—they will always remember the grace she carried into every room, the comfort she brought to every patient, and the strength she poured into every life she touched. Her legacy lives on not just in the child she helped save, but in the kindness, compassion, and quiet heroism she showed every single day of her very short career as an emergency department nurse.

Through the years afterward, Marilyn would find herself sometimes caught up in the silent aftermath of the chaos of these two tragic Saturdays in the emergency department, the sterile scent of antiseptic mingling with the lingering odor of blood and loss. The image of the heartbroken father, the shattered remains of a family, and the fading memory of her dear colleague Susan coalesced into a permanent scar—and etched deep into her soul. Every day thereafter, as she donned her scrubs, the faces of those victims and the resolute voice of her fallen friend would be with her. Those unforgettable two Saturdays, only a week apart, were not simply days marked by overwhelming tragedy; they were a bitter reminder of the fragility of life and the unyielding cost of hope in a world that sometimes refuses to grant it.

In the echoing silence of the empty ER, Marilyn vowed to carry Susan's memory with every life saved, every patient consoled, and every moment spent fighting the inevitable heartbreak of loss. And so, in the corridors of the small hospital emergency department, the heroic legacy of two nurses—one living and one lost—would forever be remembered as a testament to the valor hidden behind the everyday uniform, where even in the face of utter despair, a glimmer of humanity continued to endure.

42 BURIED STEEL

The call came in early one morning—just after shift change. EMS was inbound with a male in his late 30s experiencing what they described as "continuous seizure activity." He had no known seizure history, no meds, and no recent hospitalizations. Just a sudden onset of tonic-clonic convulsions that wouldn't stop.

The doors of the ambulance burst open as the stretcher was wheeled in. The man's body jerked violently against the straps, every muscle clenching in rhythm, saliva bubbling at the corner of his mouth. His eyes were rolled back, and he let out intermittent guttural groans between convulsions. He was posturing—rigid in some moments, flaccid in others.

Todd Clemson, ER nurse, looked up from the monitor as he slapped electrodes onto the man's chest. "Any known history of epilepsy?"

"Nope," Paramedic Herring replied. "But the family said he got into a fight last week. Refused EMS transport that night—signed a no-transport waiver. Said it was just a scalp laceration and he was not going to the hospital."

Dr. Markey, the attending ER physician, raised an eyebrow. "How bad was the cut?"

Paramedic Herring responded, "About three inches Doc. Right parietal scalp. Nothing deep, just a little bleeding."

But the way the patient was posturing told a different story.

He was intubated within minutes, and Dr. Markey ordered a full trauma panel, tox screen, head CT, and X-rays.

The X-ray tech arrived first, snapping a quick lateral skull film at bedside before whisking him off to CT. The ER team was still working on stabilizing vitals—BP was tanking, heart rate erratic, and he had a fever of 104.3.

It was Todd who first saw the film pop up on the screen.

He blinked.

"Uh... Doc? You need to see this."

Dr. Markey turned, eyes narrowing as the image loaded fully.

A long, straight, opaque foreign object extended nearly four inches into the brain cavity, beginning at the scalp wound and traveling at an angle downward and medially. There was no mistaking what it was—the unmistakable profile of a kitchen knife blade.

Perfectly intact.

Embedded in his skull.

And it had been there for a full week.

Bailey muttered under his breath, "Holy hell..."

The room fell quiet for a moment, except for the blips and beeps of monitors and the hiss of the ventilator.

Todd broke the silence. "That blade's been in there for a week?"

"Looks like it," Markey said, rubbing his forehead. "And judging by the edema, air pockets, and the fever—he's septic. Real bad."

CT only confirmed the horror. Not only was the blade buried in the brain, but a substantial abscess had formed along the trajectory, causing massive midline shift. The brain had essentially swelled around the foreign object. No external swelling. No neurological complaints—until now.

That old wound? A superficial cut on the outside. But the blade had broken off inside his skull without anyone ever knowing. And because he refused medical attention on scene, along with transport to the hospital, he was now in a very grave position.

The family—who had followed EMS in—was in disbelief. The man's brother leaned in hard against the counter in the waiting room, his voice hoarse.

"You're telling me... he had a knife in his damn head for a week?"

"Yes," Dr. Markey said, gently. "It was likely lodged during the fight, and the blade snapped. As a result of him not receiving any care initially, there was no way to know that the blade was there until now. Over time, infection set in. The seizures were his brain's response to the pressure and swelling."

The family broke down. One slammed his fist against the wall. Another sank into a chair sobbing.

Despite aggressive antibiotics, seizure control meds, and neurosurgical consultation, there was nothing that could be done.

The man coded later that night. The infection had ravaged his brain. The swelling had already begun herniating the brainstem. The knife was removed during the post-mortem—4 inches of rust-stained steel, jagged at the break.

Postscript:

In the aftermath, the story went viral through the ER. The ER staff who worked that shift still talk about it—how a man walked around with a blade in his brain and no one knew. How a fight that seemed minor was anything but. It became a cautionary tale for medics, nurses, and doctors alike: never assume the depth of a wound by the blood it spills.

Sometimes, the worst injuries are the quietest ones—buried deep, festering silently, until it's too late.

43 A JOURNEY OF COURAGE

The familiar beeping of monitors, ringing telephones, and intermittent overhead pages was part of the daily rhythm in the ER—a rhythm that seasoned nurse, Marilyn McKissack, had long since come to know by heart. But on this particular day, that rhythm was broken.

A blaring horn shattered the routine.

It was urgent. Prolonged. Not the panicked honk of someone trying to find a parking space—but the kind of sound that could shake you to your core. Marilyn's head jerked up from her charting. Before the second blast had finished, she was already heading for the ambulance bay doors.

Right on her heels was Dr. Allen Latimer, a recently recruited pulmonologist who had taken a particular interest in critical care. He was still finding his place within the emergency department's unpredictable terrain, but he had already made an impression with his calm, thoughtful approach. Marilyn had worked with dozens of doctors in her time, but something about Latimer's willingness to jump in—no matter the task—made her believe he'd last longer than most.

They pushed through the doors together and stepped into the heavy Alabama air. There, parked slightly crooked under the awning of the ambulance entrance, sat an old, dusty pickup truck. The driver's door stood ajar, the horn finally silenced. But the scene was anything but peaceful.

Behind the steering wheel was a boy—no older than ten—with wide, tear-filled eyes and trembling hands. His feet barely reached the pedals.

In the passenger seat, slumped forward onto the dashboard, was a middle-aged man, lifeless.

Marilyn didn't pause. She swung the door open, checked for signs of life, and knew immediately what she was dealing with. "He's in cardiac arrest," she said, already reaching for the seat belt.

Without hesitation, she and Dr. Latimer moved in sync, gently easing the man out of the cab and lowering him onto the sun-warmed pavement just outside the ER doors. Gravel scraped beneath their knees. Sweat already trickled down their backs. There were no crash carts, no monitors—just two medical professionals doing what they had trained their entire lives to do.

Dr. Latimer knelt beside the man, locked eyes with Marilyn, and said dryly but firmly, "I guess we're doing CPR out here, right?"

Marilyn gave a single, resolute nod. "Let's go."

And with that, compressions began.

She alternated with Latimer while barking instructions to a tech to bring out a stretcher and call for backup. Within minutes, a team came pouring through the ER doors—ER technicians, x-ray technicians, and another nurse pushing a stretcher at full speed. The body was lifted, supported by the hands of people who had long since learned to move with grace under pressure.

Inside, the code continued. The team worked the full protocol—compressions, intubation, epinephrine, defibrillation. Dr. Latimer remained focused, running the code alongside Marilyn, both of them holding on to every ounce of hope they could find. But it wasn't enough.

Eventually, time stood still in that sterile trauma bay as the final round of medications was given, the last set of compressions completed. The monitors remained flat.

Dr. Latimer glanced up at the clock and quietly called the time of death.

There was a pause, a heaviness that fell over the room like a curtain.

Marilyn stood at the head of the bed, gloved hands still at her sides, heart still racing. She hated losing them—especially the ones who made it to the doorstep, so close to help.

Later, the details emerged. The boy—whose name was Cody—had realized something was wrong with his father out in the fields of their farm, nearly 15 miles away. With no phone signal and no adults around, he had managed to hoist his unconscious father into the truck and drive—yes, drive—the entire distance to the hospital by himself. Dirt road to blacktop. Stop signs, traffic lights, and all.

He'd done it because he didn't know what else to do.

When Marilyn learned what he'd done, she had to sit down.

Marilyn looked out the window for a long moment and said. "You know, that little man did something no one will ever forget. That kid saved his father's dignity. He got him here. And sometimes, that's all we can do."

Dr. Latimer nodded. He wasn't new to medicine, but he was new to the realities of rural heartbreak. Of driveway codes. Of ten-year-old heroes.

That day became more than just a footnote in an otherwise busy shift. It became a memory etched into the fabric of the ER—proof of bravery in the unlikeliest of places, and of a boy who took the wheel when it mattered most.

More than forty years have passed since that day in the ambulance bay—the day a dusty pickup truck pulled up with a boy behind the wheel and a dying man in the passenger seat. For many, it became just another story whispered in hospital hallways, a tale told to new staff to remind them of the unpredictability and raw humanity of emergency medicine.

But for Dr. Allen Latimer and Marilyn McKissack, it was never just a story. It was a turning point.

Soon after this case, the hospital moved to a new location. Today, you will find that Dr. Latimer is still walking those halls with a quiet authority that commands both trust and admiration. He serves as an intensivist on the critical care team, where the most complex and fragile patients are placed in his care. Though time has etched some lines into his face and slowed his gait just a little, his mind remains sharp, his instincts honed, and his compassion as steadfast as ever.

He is a man who has not only seen the evolution of medicine but helped shape it. Students seek him out for guidance. Nurses breathe easier when he's on the floor. Families cling to his words, knowing they are spoken not just with knowledge but with heart. He is respected by all who know him—not because of the titles he's earned or the cases he's conquered, but because of how he's always shown up: steady, calm, and ready to do the work.

Marilyn was right all those years ago when she looked at the fresh-faced pulmonologist and silently decided he had what it took.

"He's going to be around a while," she had told a coworker that evening, long after the code had ended and the ER had settled back into its rhythm.

She wasn't wrong.

Dr. Latimer never forgot Marilyn either—her grit, her grace, and her instinct to lead with heart. Though she eventually retired, her legacy lives on in stories like that driveway code, and in the lives of patients she touched—and in doctors like Latimer, who still carry her lessons in their every move.

Some stories in the ER fade over time. But the best ones—the real ones—become part of its foundation. And sometimes, if you're lucky, the heroes from those stories are still walking the halls, still answering the call, and still saving lives.

Just like Dr. Allen Latimer.

44 Church Choir & Oxy

It was just after shift change on a Tuesday morning—typically a short period of about 45 minutes each day that offered a lull in the ER's chaos. The fluorescent lights buzzed overhead, casting their usual sterile glow across half-empty rooms and a fresh new staff. That peaceful rhythm, however, was short-lived.

"Through the double doors came a sound we all recognized long before we saw her", said Meghan Cole, ER Charge Nurse.

"*OHHHHHH LORD HAVE MERCY, I'M IN PAIN!*"

There she was—Loretta Jane Delrose. A frequent flyer, a regular on the ER bingo card of chaos, and a self-declared "pain management specialist" with a unique knack for dramatics. She was wheeled in by security—again—legs flailing, arms twitching, and her voice echoing through the halls like a Pentecostal revival gone sideways.

"I NEED THREE PERCOCET! THREE! THAT'S ALL I'M ASKIN' FOR!" she wailed, clutching her abdomen one second, then her lower back the next, then just waving her hands toward the heavens as if asking God Himself to drop the pills into her lap.

Meghan, was a seasoned charge nurse with a steel spine and sarcasm sharper than a scalpel, raised an eyebrow and muttered, “Well, praise Jesus—she’s back.”

Loretta was taken to Room 6, the usual spot. As the door closed behind them, the show began in full force. She rolled back and forth on the stretcher like it was a canoe in a hurricane, letting out moans that made some of the young nursing students blush. She kicked the bed rails, pounded the mattress, and called out to each nurse who passed by:

“Hey baby, I’m clean now! Just three Percocet and I’ll be good as new. That ain’t too much to ask!”

Dr. Andrew Johns entered the room—a stoic ER physician with a dry wit and zero patience for games. He stood just inside the room, arms crossed, as Loretta launched into her latest performance.

"Doc, listen to me. I'm not the same woman I used to be. I've been goin' to church every Sunday. I gave my life to Jesus. I don't do drugs no more. I'm clean. Clean as a whistle. I just need my medicine for the pain, and I swear, just three Percocet, that's all!"

Dr. Johns looked at her with an expression of frustration and replied, "Three Percocet, huh? Just three?"

She nodded feverishly.

He paused for a moment, then shrugged. "Alright. I'll write you a script for three—*if* you can sing one part of a church hymn that you sing at your new church."

She stopped mid-writhing and blinked at him. "Say what?"

"You heard me," he said, arms still folded. "Sing me a line from a hymn. Prove you're really going to church."

Without hesitation, she sat bolt upright in the bed like she'd been resurrected from the grave and belted out:

"NOTHING BUT THE BLOOD OF JESUS..."

Then immediately added,

"NOW GIVE ME MY DAMN PERCOCET!"

A stunned silence fell for a split second—then the hallway erupted. Meghan nearly dropped her clipboard. One of the techs snorted so hard he nearly choked. A nursing student standing nearby whispered, "Did that *just* happen?"

Dr. Johns, doing his best to keep a straight face, slowly turned around and walked out of the room shaking his head. "I'll write for two," he muttered.

Loretta was eventually discharged, still humming gospel hymns as she left the building—prescription in hand, victory in her step, and the Spirit of the Lord (or something stronger) all over her. Miraculously her pain was gone!

And from that day forward, Room 6 wasn't just a room.

It was a stage.

And Loretta? She was the star of the only show where pain management met Sunday morning choir practice.

45 Dead or Alive

The midmorning lull had settled over the ER like a soft blanket—brief, fragile, and soon to be disturbed. Burl Williams, the emergency department technician, stood near the ambulance bay doors sipping from a coffee cup he'd been microwaving and re-microwaving since 6 a.m. Known to everyone simply as Burl, he was a short man with white hair and a white mustache, slow drawl, and a work ethic built like a cinder block wall—solid, dependable, and immovable.

Burl didn't rush to do anything. He didn't need to. In fact, his slow, deliberate movements had become part of the rhythm of the ER itself. Staff would joke, "If Burl's moving' fast, somebody better check the weather in hell." But no one questioned his dedication. He showed up early, stayed late, and helped wherever he was needed. Whether someone needed a wheelchair ride to X-ray or a body moved to the morgue, Burl handled it all—with the same steady pace and a quiet sense of duty.

That morning, a security officer knocked on the bay doors, waving toward a beat-up Buick idling just outside. Burl shuffled out to investigate. Inside the car was an older man in his late sixties, slumped slightly in the front seat. A younger man—his son, maybe—looked panicked.

"Hey, I think he's sick or somethin'... can y'all get him inside?"

Without a word, Burl opened the passenger door, slid a wheelchair into place, and with gentle effort, loaded the man into it. The man did not move, his arms hung strangely stiff, but Burl thought maybe he was just unconscious—or maybe postictal from a seizure. He'd seen stranger things in his time. One thing was for sure, he wasn't going to leave the man out there in the summer heat.

"Let's get you a room," Burl mumbled under his breath, half to himself, half to the unmoving patient.

He rolled the man inside, passing slowly by the nurses' station. The wheels of the chair squeaked softly, like they too were in no rush. Nurses watched him pass as if it were a funeral procession.

"There goes Burl," one nurse whispered. "In no great hurry."

Burl continued past two open exam rooms—Rooms 1 and 2—both clean and ready. But he had his mind set on Room 3. Room 3 had a functioning oxygen wall hookup, a stocked cabinet, and it was next to the crash cart—just in case. Never mind the fact that the man hadn't moved an inch or made a sound. Burl followed protocol. Everyone got a room. Period.

He positioned the wheelchair next to the bed in Room 3 and began the awkward dance of transferring the man. It was then that something seemed...off. The man's arms didn't flop naturally. His legs didn't bend when Burl tried to lift them. In fact, they didn't move at all.

Burl paused, squinting at the man's face. His eyes were partially open but glazed. There was no chest rise. No warmth. No pulse. No breath. Just a vacant stare and a body as stiff as a board.

Burl stepped out into the hallway and waved casually at the nurse's desk. "Room 3's gonna need a nurse," he called out, as calm as ever.

When two nurses entered the room moments later, what they found stopped them cold. The man wasn't in need of care—he was long past it. His skin was pale and cool, mottled with lividity. His limbs were fixed in rigor mortis. There was no emergency to treat. Only the realization that this man had been dead—completely and unmistakably dead—before he ever rolled through the ER doors.

The charge nurse turned to Burl, her mouth slightly open. "Burl ... this man is... he's dead. He's been dead for a while."

Burl blinked once, nodded slowly, and replied, "Well, I figured somethin' wasn't quite right. But I wasn't gonna leave him out in that heat. Dead or alive, everyone deserves a room."

And that was Burl in a nutshell. Unflappable, respectful, and methodical to the core. Word of the incident spread quickly through the ER, and by lunch, staff were already telling the story between sips of sweet tea and bites of vending machine chips.

"Only Burl," someone laughed, "would treat a dead guy like he had a ten-minute wait time."

The man was later identified by his son, and his family confirmed he'd been having chest pain the night before shortly before he went to bed. They found him like this that morning when he did not get up for breakfast. They decided to load him in the vehicle themselves and rush him to the ER instead of calling 911. But thanks to Burl, he wasn't left slumped over in a car seat, baking in the Alabama sun. He was wheeled in with quiet dignity—stiff, yes, but never ignored.

Over the years, his co-workers would make jokes about it, but Burl never let them bother him. He'd just smile, sip his coffee, and roll on to the next job—slow and steady, just the way he always did.

Because in Burl's ER, everyone got a room. Dead or alive.

46 The Gospel According to Daren

Some nights in the ER feel like you're swimming upstream with a bag of bricks strapped to your back—and this was one of those nights. "We were getting our collective asses handed to us: traumas stacked up, psych holds overflowing, call bells ringing like we were hosting a game show, and a charge nurse muttering in tongues," said ER nurse, Steve Hartman.

Triage was bursting at the seams, and he was trying to help clear the bottleneck. That's when he got called to assess a new arrival—an 18-year-old male with what was listed as a "possible ankle sprain."

Simple enough, he thought.

Steve stepped into triage to find a grown man—technically an adult—sitting in a wheelchair, wailing like he'd been shot. His right ankle was swollen, sure, but no bone sticking out, no deformity. He was holding his leg like it had been amputated mid-field.

Hovering over him was his mother, gently stroking his hair and whispering, "It's okay, baby. You're so strong."

Strong?

Across from them stood Dad. Red-faced, slurring slightly, reeking of whiskey and indignation. His words came out with all the charm of a drunk at a wedding toast gone wrong.

"I *demand* an orthopedic surgeon be called. Right NOW," the dad said.

Steve calmly explained that he'd be seen by the ER physician first, and if ortho was needed, they'd be consulted. That's how it works.

Dad didn't like that.

He *really* didn't like it when he was told that there was not a room available, and they'd have to wait in the lobby.

He gave Steve a stare that might've worked on someone less caffeinated and sleep-deprived.

"You'll regret this," he mumbled as they wheeled out to wait.

About fifteen minutes later, a room finally opened up. They got the young man back—still crying, still being petted like a nervous cat—and placed them in an exam room.

Steve was charting at the nurses' station when he saw movement in his peripheral vision. And then—**stomp stomp**—here came Dad.

He was marching up the hallway like he'd been summoned to the battlefield, face flushed, chest puffed, fists already clenched with righteous fury.

He stopped right at the station, leaned in, and growled:

"You people need to understand—there's *another* hospital in this town we can go to."

Hartman didn't blink. "I'm aware of that," He replied flatly. "And you're free to leave at any time if that's what you choose."

He didn't appreciate Steve's calm tone.

He stepped further into the nurses' station—**a big no-no**—and hissed, "I don't need your attitude. You're about a smartass. You may be *fixin'* to get your ass whipped."

Steve said, "Let me be clear—I've had threats before. Comes with the territory. But there was something about the way he said it—eyes glassy, lip curled—that made me know he thought he was about to deliver some backwoods justice."

So Steve looked him square in the eye and said, calmly:

"I might."

Pause.

"And I might not."

That was enough to freeze the air in the room. Visitors started drifting out of their rooms like moths to a porchlight. One leaned against the doorway, arms crossed like he was about to enjoy some prime entertainment.

Another ER nurse was whispering, "Sir, please, go back to your room."

"No," he said, eyes fixed on them. "I want to *see* it when that big guy gets enough and stomps that drunk man's ass."

The tension could've been cut with trauma shears.

Finally, the dad muttered something under his breath and stormed back toward the lobby. The spell was broken, and people slowly returned to their rooms, disappointed that the bout was called before the first bell.

One of the bystanders—middle-aged guy in khakis and a polo—walked up to the station, pulled a business card from his wallet, and handed it to Steve.

"If you catch any crap over this," he said, "tell them to call me. You showed remarkable restraint."

Steve just smiled politely. "I appreciate that. He's just worried about his son."

The man shook his head. "No excuse. That was unacceptable."

A few weeks later, Steve and his wife at the time, decided they needed to "get involved" and try out one of the larger churches in town. She'd heard good things. They got dressed up, shook off the night shift fatigue, and went to visit.

They walked into the sanctuary, then down the hall to their assigned Sunday school class. The room was bright, warm, and smelled of coffee and baked goods. People were chatting in polite southern tones. It felt... safe.

Until the door opened, and in walked the teacher.

Red-faced Dad.

He smiled warmly at the class as he grabbed a Bible and said, "Alright y'all, let's open in prayer."

Steve leaned over and whispered to his wife: "We... cannot stay in this class."

"Why not?"

"Because that man," he said, pointing subtly with my chin, "was drunk in the ER a few weeks ago and threatened to whip my ass."

They didn't go back.

Steve said, "Because as much as I believe in forgiveness, grace, and turning the other cheek... I also believe in *not* getting glared at during Sunday school while flipping through the Book of Matthew."

EPILOGUE/CONCLUSION

Emergency medicine is a world of extremes—life and death, chaos and calm, heartbreak and hope. The stories in this book offer just a glimpse into the reality faced by the nurses and physicians who dedicate their lives to this work each day. They are the ones who run toward the crisis, who hold the hands of the suffering and dying, who make incredibly important decisions in the blink of an eye.

But what happens after the adrenaline fades away, after the shift ends? The aftermath is different for each of them. Some carry their losses home like a shadow, others find comfort in the lives they saved. Some learn to compartmentalize, to separate the personal from the professional. And yet, no one emerges unchanged. Every patient leaves an imprint on your mind, every case becomes a lesson, and every moment in the ER shapes the next.

Despite the exhaustion, the heartbreak, and the sacrifices that are made, these nurses and doctors come back shift after shift. They do it because someone has to do it. Because on the worst day of your life, you need someone who won't give up on you.

This book is not just about medicine—it's about humanity. It's about resilience, compassion, and the unwavering commitment of those who stand on the frontlines. And though the stories may end here, the work continues, the lives saved and lost remain in their hearts, and the aftermath is never really truly over.

For every ER nurse and physician in the trenches—you are seen, you are valued, and the world is a better place because of you. Thank you for doing what you do!

May God bless you and forever keep you safe.

BIBLIOGRAPHY

Quote by William Osler – "A good doctor treats the disease; a great doctor treats the patient who has the disease." - William Osler

Green, Reg. *The Nicholas Effect.* Reg Green Publications. January 15, 2021.

Hall, Jimmy. *Rekindled – True Stories of the Fire and EMS.* HammerTyme Books. March 1, 2025.

Suicide Prevention Center Life Line-July 16, 2022 Retrieved from https://suicidepreventionlifeline.org/current-events/the-lifeline-and-988/

African Proverb – "When an old man dies, a library burns to the ground." — Amadou Hampâté Bâ

"Greater love has no one than this, than to lay down one's life for his friends." —*John 15:13 (NKJV)*

ACKNOWLEDGMENTS

Throughout my career in fire, EMS, and nursing, I've often heard people say, "You guys should write a book!" Like many of you, I considered it, but my motivation never quite reached the level needed to turn that idea into reality.

Then, midway through the COVID-19 pandemic, I found myself attending the funerals of many close friends and colleagues. It was during this difficult time that I realized the importance of moving forward with this project.

"When an old man dies,

a library burns to the ground."

African Proverb- Amadou Hampâté Bâ

With each passing, a lifetime of wisdom, experiences, and stories vanishes—often unheard and unrecorded. We recognized that the voices of our brothers and sisters should not fade into history but instead be preserved and shared for future generations to come.

The loss of a very close brother, Chuck Crawford, only reinforced what I had already come to realize—the time for preservation is now. In June of 2021, Chuck and I began assembling the thoughts in our heads for this project. Unfortunately, a few months later, before we could get started, he too left. And with him, a lifetime of stories!

This book is a testament to the good, the bad, and the ugly—capturing the stories that define our shared experiences from the emergency department arena. Tomorrow is never promised to us, which is why our mission must be fulfilled today.

I am incredibly proud to present *Aftermath in the ER* and equally as proud to have worked alongside some of the most skilled, knowledgeable, and selfless healthcare professionals throughout my career. Thank you for your time, your expertise, and, most of all, for the unwavering force that binds us together.

LIST OF CONTRIBUTORS

Marilyn McKissack, RN

Chris Hovey, RN

"Shelley Mae", RN

"Hazel Ray", RN

Amanda Caples, RN

Meghan Cole, CRNP

Dr. Allen Latimer, Pulmonologist / Intensivist

Zack Marden, RN

Steve Hartman, RN

Tim Adamcryk, ER MD

Cade Hall, ER Tech

Jeanne Emrick, RN

Robert Smith, RN

Amanda Powers, RN

Loving Remembrance of Some Great Heroes

Dale Shaw

Thomas Rose

Mark & Judy Howell

Janie Powell

Terry Olive

Ray Griffin

Susan Deal

William Lupinacci

Russell Page

Carl Barlow

Jerry Hope

Chuck Crawford

Christy Edwards

Peggy Spiliotis

Earl Burke

About the Author

Jimmy Hall's extensive career in emergency services, nursing, and education has profoundly impacted the Dothan, Alabama, community. His dedication to fire, medical, and nursing services, combined with his commitment to training future professionals, exemplifies his significant influence on public safety and healthcare.

Career Highlights:

- **Fire Service:** Jimmy began his career as a Fire Medic with the Dothan Fire Department, later advancing to the role of Fire Sergeant Engineer with the department's inaugural truck company. His leadership and technical expertise were instrumental in the department's operations.
- **Emergency Medical Services (EMS):** With over two decades of experience as a Nationally Registered Emergency Medical Technician-Paramedic (NREMTP), Jimmy served with local EMS agencies,

including Pilcher Ambulance Service. His dedication to patient care and emergency response was widely recognized.

- **Education and Training:** As an instructor for the EMS program at a local college, Jimmy taught EMT and paramedic classes, along with specialized rescue training courses such as High Angle Rope Rescue, Vehicle Rescue and Extrication, Interior Search and Rescue, and Water Rescue. His commitment to education has shaped many professionals in the field.
- **Certifications and Achievements:** Jimmy holds numerous certifications in specialized rescue, Fire & EMS Instruction, Hydraulics and Pump Operation, and HazMat Operations. He has completed multiple courses in the fire science curriculum and holds double Associate Degrees in EMS and Nursing. His dedication to excellence was recognized in 1994 when he received a certificate of heroism from the city commission for his role in a high-angle water tank rescue. In 1995, he was

honored as the Paramedic of the Year by Flowers Hospital.

- **Current Role:** Jimmy currently serves as a Board Certified Vascular Access Nurse at a local hospital, continuing his commitment to healthcare and patient well-being.

Personal Life:

Residing in Dothan, Alabama, Jimmy enjoys life with his wife, Pam, their sons Seth and Cade, and their four-legged daughter, Zoey.

www.ingramcontent.com/pod-product-compliance
Lightning Source LLC
LaVergne TN
LVHW100301210926
848480LV00003B/991